Bill 'Swampy' Marsh is an award-winning writer/performer of stories, songs and plays. He spent most of his youth in rural south-western New South Wales. Bill was forced to give up any idea he had of a 'career' as a cricketer when a stint at agricultural college was curtailed because of illness, and so began his hobby of writing. After backpacking through three continents and working in the wine industry, his writing hobby blossomed into a career.

His first collection of short stories, *Beckom Pop. 64*, was published in 1988, his second, *Old Yanconian Daze*, in 1995 and his third, *Looking for Dad*, in 1998. During 1999 Bill released *Australia*, a CD of songs and stories. That was followed in 2002 by *A Drover's Wife* and *Glory, Glory—A Tribute to the Royal Flying Doctor Service*, in 2008. He has written soundtrack songs and music for the television documentaries *The Last Mail from Birdsville—The Story of Tom Kruse*, *Source to Sea—The Story of the Murray Riverboats* and the German travel documentary *Traumzeit auf dem Stuart Highway*.

Bill runs writing workshops in schools and communities and is a teacher of short story writing within the Adelaide

Institute of TAFE's Professional Writing Unit. He has won and judged many nationwide short story writing and songwriting competitions and short film awards.

New Great Australian Flying Doctor Stories is Bill's third book of Flying Doctor stories and is part of a very successful series of his 'Great Australian' stories, including: *The ABC Book of Great Aussie Stories for Young People* (2010), *Great Australian Stories—Outback Towns and Pubs* (2009), *More Great Australian Flying Doctor Stories* (2007), *Great Australian Railway Stories* (2005), *Great Australian Droving Stories* (2003) *Great Australian Shearing Stories* (2001) and *Great Australian Flying Doctor Stories* (1999). Bill's story of *Goldie* was published in 2008.

More information about the author can be found at www.billswampymarsh.com

New Great Australian
FLYING
DOCTOR
STORIES

New Great Australian
FLYING DOCTOR STORIES

Bill 'Swampy' Marsh

ABC
Books

Publisher's note: The stories contained in this compilation are derived from interviews. In order to preserve the authenticity of these oral accounts the language used is faithful to the original story-telling. The publisher does not necessarily endorse the views expressed or the language used in any of the stories.

Warning: This book may contain the names of Aboriginal and Torres Strait Islander people now deceased.

The ABC 'Wave' device is a trademark of the Australian Broadcasting Corporation and is used under licence by HarperCollins*Publishers* Australia.

First published in Australia in 2010
by HarperCollins*Publishers* Australia Pty Limited
ABN 36 009 913 517
harpercollins.com.au

Quotation on page 151 from *From the City to the Sandhills of Birdsville*, by Mona Henry, reproduced by permission of CopyRight Publishing.
Quotations on pages 202–207 from *Outback Achiever: Fred McKay—Successor to Flynn of the Inland*, by Maisie McKenzie, reproduced by permission of Boolarong Press.
Lyrics from 'Woman on the Land', on page 114, written by John Williamson © 1977 Emusic Pty. Limited, reproduced by permission.

HarperCollins*Publishers*
25 Ryde Road, Pymble, Sydney, NSW 2073, Australia
31 View Road, Glenfield, Auckland 0627, New Zealand
A 53, Sector 57, Noida, UP, India
77–85 Fulham Palace Road, London W6 8JB, United Kingdom
2 Bloor Street East, 20th floor, Toronto, Ontario M4W 1A8, Canada
10 East 53rd Street, New York NY 10022, USA

National Library of Australia Cataloguing-in-Publication data:

Marsh, Bill, 1950-
  New great Australian flying doctor stories / Bill Marsh.
  978 0 7333 2551 9 (pbk.)
  Royal Flying Doctor Service of Australia.
  Aeronautics in medicine—Australia.
362.1042570994

Cover design by Priscilla Nielsen
Cover image © Kit Kittle/CORBIS
Typeset in 10.5/18pt ITC Bookman Light by Kirby Jones
Printed and bound in Australia by Griffin Press
70gsm Classic White used by HarperCollins*Publishers* is a natural, recyclable product made from wood grown in sustainable forests. The manufacturing processes conform to the environmental regulations in the country of origin, Finland.

5 4 3 2 1   10 11 12 13

To Howard William Steer

—with many thanks for all your help and great spirit

www.howardsteerart.com.au

Contents

Contributors

New Great Australian Flying Doctor Stories is based on stories told to Bill 'Swampy' Marsh by:

Rhonda Anstee

Bob Balmain

Rod Bishop

Paul Brady

Chris Carter

Donna Cattanach

Jane Clemson

Ruth Cook

Dave Crommelin

Heather Curtin

Phil and Sue Darby

Sarah Fenton

Richard Fewster and Ann
   Ruston

Norton Gill

Jack Goldsmith

David Hansford

Wal 'Dusty' Harkness

David and Christine Harris

Robina Jeffs

Ruth Ko

Margaret Loveday

John Lynch

Susan Markwell

Bill 'Swampy' Marsh

Neil McDougall

David McInnes

Ian 'Mac' McKechnie

Barbara Meredith

Kevin Murphy

Shirley Norris

Stephen Penberthy

Peter Phillips

Bill Rawson

Cheryl Russ

Chris Smith

Howard William Steer

Kim Tyrie

Esther Veldstra

Nick Watling

Margaret Wheatley

Margaret Worth

A Brief History

On a number of occasions people have mentioned that while they've greatly enjoyed the collected stories of the Royal Flying Doctor Service (RFDS), there's never been the one story that gives a brief overview as to just how the RFDS came into being. For me, history isn't just a list of dates that relate to a sequence of events. I had enough of that back in school. But since then I've developed a great interest in the many and varied characters who have been involved in the making of our history: people like the shearers and the drovers, those who have worked and travelled on our railways, those who live and work in little outback towns and pubs.

The RFDS has been, and still is, full of people who are prepared to take on the huge challenges that working our outback regions presents, and for the betterment of all. As one person I interviewed for *More Great Flying Doctor Stories* said, those who are involved in the Flying Doctor Service, 'on a daily basis put their lives on the line for people who are complete strangers to them. They don't care who these people are or what their nationality or religion is. And it doesn't matter [that] those very same people probably wouldn't take a similar risk for them. In fact they wouldn't even realise the risk. What's more, the RFDS do it for free.'

So where did this amazing organisation have its origins? Who were the driving forces behind its conception? What sort of characters were they? Well, to begin at the beginning, the Reverend John Flynn was the person who had the dream of creating a spiritual and medical 'mantle of safety' for all remote and outback people, regardless of colour, race or creed. And what a large dream it was. As Hudson Fysh, the co-founder of Qantas, once wrote of John Flynn: 'Flynn the Dreamer ... who saw a vision of a Flying Doctor well before the days of practical flying, but kept it firmly fixed in his mind.'

John Flynn was born in the late 1880s, at a place called Moliagul in central-western Victoria. He went to a few primary schools, one of which had the rather uninviting name of Snake Valley. In 1898 he matriculated from high school; then, to help pay his way through his further education, he became what was called a 'pupil-teacher' with the Victorian Education Department. Following that he began training for the ministry. His time at theological college was broken up by two important events that ignited his passion for the bush and its people; the first being the couple of periods he spent on a shearers' mission and stemming from those experiences was the publication of his *Bushman's Companion*.

After being ordained in 1911 John Flynn volunteered to go to the Smith of Dunesk Mission, at Beltana, in the remote northern Flinders Ranges of South Australia. Dunesk had been established by the Presbyterian Church and was located in a parish that covered a vast area of the South Australian inland that extended over to the railhead at Oodnadatta.

Oodnadatta was situated along the original old Ghan railway line and at that time it had a floating population of around a hundred or so. Many were Aboriginal, plus there were the Afghan traders—hence the term 'the Ghan'. Oodnadatta also happens to be one of the hottest places in Australia, with temperatures of over fifty degrees celsius having been recorded.

Anyway, that's where the mission had placed a nursing sister and where it had also planned to build a nursing hostel, and it was under Flynn's guidance that the Oodnadatta Nursing Hostel was opened in late 1911. The following year the church asked Flynn to survey the Northern Territory region and after he handed in a couple of reports—one on the needs of Aborigines and the other on the needs of white settlers—the Presbyterian General Assembly appointed him as superintendent of what was to be named the Australian Inland Mission (AIM). In doing so the South Australian, Western Australian and Queensland assemblies transferred their remote areas into Flynn's care. So the AIM was officially established and it commenced operations out of Oodnadatta with just the one hostel, the one nursing sister, the one padre and a 'fleet' of five camels. It began, as it has continued, 'without preference for nationality or creed', and was based on the idea of a remote areas network of nursing hostels and hospitals, all working in conjunction with a patrol padre.

By 1918, and despite World War I, John Flynn had managed to establish patrol padres out of Port Hedland and Broome in Western Australia, Pine Creek in the Northern

Territory and Cloncurry in Queensland. He'd also appointed
nursing sisters to Port Hedland and Halls Creek in Western
Australia, and to Maranboy and Alice Springs in the Northern
Territory.

Flynn's commitment to the AIM was absolute. He even
involved himself in the design of the nursing hostels, along
with the architects, engineers and the local people. His
aim was to make sure that each building suited its own
particular regional climatic conditions and the availability of
local building material. The large stone building of the Alice
Springs Hostel is such an example. He helped design it in
such a way that it was cooled via a tunnel under the ground
floor, where wet bags filtered the dust, and then the cooled air
was drawn, by convection, through the hostel wards. Then as
the air heated up it rose to the lantern roof from where it was
expelled. Wide verandahs also provided extra cooling.

Another of Flynn's passions was his magazine, the
Inlander. The *Inlander* was used to spread the word to a
wider Australian public. This was where he first mentioned
his idea of a 'mantle of safety'. The magazine also promoted
his fight for a 'brighter bush' with his photographs,
documents, statistics, maps and articles telling of the needs
of the outback people. He also wrote about inland Australia's
potential for development and about how it could only reach
its full potential by providing for the women and children.
He didn't overlook the Aborigines either. And, mind you,
there weren't too many people around back then who were
as outspoken or knowledgeable as Flynn was on the subject.

In fact, one particular issue of a 1915 *Inlander* was pretty much entirely devoted to the plight of the 'fringe-dwellers' and described how their situation was 'a blot on Australia'. He went on to say, 'We who so cheerfully sent a cheque for £100,000 to Belgium to help a people pushed out of their own inheritance by foreigners ... surely we must just as cheerfully do something for those whom we clean-handed people have dispossessed in the interests of superior culture.'

The next part of Flynn's overall strategy of a mantle of safety was focused on the possibility of radio communications between doctor and patient and the idea of a 'Flying Doctor'. In Flynn's mind the two had to work hand-in-hand. Even as early as 1925 he said that 'the practicability of the Flying Doctor proposal depends almost entirely on the widespread adoption of wireless by bush residents'.

To that end, in late May 1925, Flynn and a returned soldier and radio technician by the name of George Towns took delivery of a specially designed Dodge Buckboard that was to be used for the first inland experiments in radio transmission. They picked the vehicle up in Adelaide and drove to Alice Springs via Beltana, Innamincka, Birdsville, Marree and Oodnadatta, doing test transmissions as they went. Interestingly enough, they used a pulley drive from the jacked-up back wheel of the Dodge to generate electricity for radio transmission.

The following year the ever-persuasive Flynn talked a man called Alfred Traeger into going to Alice Springs to conduct further experiments. Alf Traeger was to become another vital link in the development of the Flying Doctor Service. Alf was born near Dimboola, Victoria, back in the late 1800s. I guess if he lived today Alf Traeger might be considered a bit of a geek. He was once described as 'a curious, patient, precise child, who, at twelve, made a telephone receiver and transmitted between the toolshed and his house'. So it seems his pathway in life was set very early on.

After his parents had moved to South Australia, Alf attended Balaklava Public School and the Martin Luther School before going to a technical high school. He then studied mechanical and electrical engineering before being employed by the Metropolitan Tramways Trust and the Postmaster-General's Department. When World War I started he tried to enlist but was refused on the grounds of his Germanic heritage, this is even though his grandparents had been naturalised. For Alf, not to be able to serve his country was one of his bitter disappointments.

Instead, Alf threw himself into his work and it wasn't long after he'd obtained an amateur operator's licence and built his first pedal transmitter-receiver that he formed Traeger Transceivers Pty Ltd. That's when John Flynn arrived on the scene and employed Alf to help him out. After a brief outback tour where it's said that despite the severe heat Alf always wore a dark suit and braces, he returned to Adelaide to start developing a transceiver for the Flying Doctor network.

Flynn's basic outline to Traeger was simple: these radio sets had to be cheap, durable, small and easy to operate. So by using bicycle pedals to drive the generator, Alf found that a person could comfortably achieve 20 watts at a pressure of about 300 volts. He then enclosed the generator's fly-wheel and gears in a metal housing, with the pedals outside, and added a cast base so that the whole contraption could be screwed to the floor beneath a table. Traeger built the transceiver into a box, and set up a master switch to separate the crystal controller transmitter from the receiver. To put it more simply, Traeger's wireless was basically a pedal-operated generator, which provided power for a transceiver. But as simple as it seems, once the first pedal sets came on the market in the late-1920s they created a communications revolution, especially throughout the remote inland.

While Traeger was working on his pedal wireless, Flynn had been busy on the second part of his overall strategy, and that was to try to set up an aerial medical service. Some say that Flynn's original vision of a 'flying doctor' had been inspired by a letter from a Lieutenant John Clifford Peel—or just Clifford Peel, as he preferred to be known. Now, going back to around 1912, a then eighteen-year-old Clifford Peel had read a book John Flynn had written, titled *Northern Territory and Central Australia: A Call to the Church*. Apparently the book captured Peel's interest in the work Flynn was doing and the problems he faced of being able to cover the huge distances he needed to, to create his mantle of safety. The book got Peel thinking about the logistics of how aerial care could be provided to the people in the remote areas of Australia.

Then, later on, after World War I began, Peel trained as a pilot at Laverton in Victoria. The story goes that he wrote to

Flynn with some of the thoughts he had on the practicalities of using aeroplanes within the AIM. Now, keep it in mind that, back then, aeroplanes were a relatively new invention and, to the vast majority of people it would seem bonkers to jump into a basic wooden frame with a bit of canvas stretched over it and go flying into the vast unknown of outback Australia. But the idea excited Flynn. He wanted more information, which in turn produced Peel's much recorded reply of November 1917. At the time the letter was written, Peel was sailing from Melbourne to the United Kingdom, on his way to begin his life as a wartime airman. In part, it read:

Aviation is still new, but it has set some of us thinking, and thinking hard. Perhaps others want to be thinking too. Hence these few notes.

Safety.

The first question to be asked is sure to be 'Is it safe?'

To the Australian lay mind the thought of flying is accompanied by many weird ideas of its danger. True there are dangers, which in the Inland will be accompanied by the possibility of being stranded in the desert without food or water. Yet even with this disadvantage the only reply to such a query is a decided affirmative. Practically all the flying for the last three years has been military flying ... and if we study the records available ... we will find that the number of miles flown per misadventure is very large, while the number of accidents per aerodrome per annum is very small.

Difficulties.

As in every new adventure there are initial difficulties ... The first and greatest of these is cost ... With aeroplanes I venture to say that, given proper care, the upkeep is relatively light while the cost of installing compares very favourably if we realise that to run a train, motor car, lorry, or other vehicle, roads must first be made and then kept in repair, whilst the air needs no such preparation.

The problem of overhauls and major repairs present another great difficulty ... The question of ways and means remains to be solved. Landing grounds may present some difficulties in certain regions, but these will be found where needed. Machines for Inland work will need to have a large radius of action, say a non-stop run of at least 700 miles, so that the fuel carrying capacity will be large.

Many of these and other difficulties loom very large, as we view them from the distance, but with the progress of aviation, and the more universal use of the motor car, many of them will automatically disappear.

Advantages.

The advantage of an air service will be quickly appreciated ... With a machine doing 90 miles an hour, Darwin is brought within twelve and a half hours of Oodnadatta (excluding stops). It takes little imagination to see the advantage of this to the mail service, government officials, and business men while to the frontier settlers it will be an undreamt of boon as regards household supplies, medical attention, and business.

A Scheme.

Just by way of a suggestive scheme, I propose to consider that portion of A.I.M. territory east of the Western Australian boundary. In this large tract of land, consisting of one-third of the Australian continent, I am assuming that the bases are situated at Oodnadatta in South Australia, Cloncurry in Queensland and Katherine in the Northern Territory. At the present time these are railheads, hence supplies can be brought up with comparative regularity and minimum cost. From each of these centres the A.I.M. workers can work a district of say 300 miles radius, or an area of 270,000 square miles.

In the not very distant future, if our church folk only realise the need, I can see a missionary doctor administering to the needs of men and women scattered between Wyndham and Cloncurry, Darwin and Hergott [now named Marree]. If the nation can do so much in the days of war surely it will do its 'bit' in the coming days of peace—and here is its chance.

The credit side of the ledger I leave for those interested in the development of our hinterland to compute. Sufficient to say that the heroes of the Inland are laying the foundation stones of our Australian nation.

> J.CLIFFORD PEEL, LIEUT
> Australian Flying Corps, A.I.F.
> At Sea, 20/11/17.

Unfortunately, Peel didn't live to see just how successful his idea became because only thirteen months later—and only seven weeks before the end of the war—his aircraft disappeared during a routine patrol in France. The mystery of Peel's fate has never been solved. But the seeds had been sown.

How those seeds grew to fruition came about through Flynn's friendship with two men: Sir W. Hudson Fysh and Hugh Victor McKay.

Hudson Fysh was born in the mid-1890s at Launceston, Tasmania. It doesn't appear that he was the most dedicated of students because, after attending various schools, he went out working as a jackeroo and wool classer. When World War I started he enlisted in the Australian Light Horse Brigade and served at Gallipoli and in Egypt and Palestine. He was commissioned lieutenant in 1916. Following that he transferred to the Australian Flying Corps where he won the Distinguished Flying Cross.

After the war Fysh and another ex-serviceman, Pat McGinness, along with Arthur Baird, an engineer, decided to enter the Australian government's £10,000-prize contest for a flight from England to Australia. But because of the death of their backer, Sir Samuel McCaughey, that didn't happen.

Instead, Fysh and McGinness were paid by the government to survey the Longreach to Darwin section of the contest route. They did this in the first vehicle to go overland to the Gulf of Carpentaria, a Model T Ford.

The next year Fysh and McGinness, along with three Queensland graziers, got together and formed the Queensland and Northern Territory Aerial Services Ltd, or Qantas, as it's known these days. With only an Avro Dyak and an old BE2E war-disposals aircraft, the company moved from Winton to Longreach where the planes were then used as a taxi service, as an ambulance, for stock inspection services and for joy-riding. Around about this time Hudson Fysh and John Flynn struck up a friendship and they talked about the practicalities and possibilities of a Flying Doctor Service. In doing so, Fysh told Flynn that he'd be willing to support him in any way he could.

Hugh Victor McKay was another person who helped John Flynn create a Flying Doctor Service. Hugh McKay was born at Raywood, Victoria, in the mid 1860s. He was the fifth of twelve children and he had very little education other than his parents' devotion to the Bible. By the age of thirteen he was working on the farm.

Back in those days harvesting was done with a horse-drawn stripper and manual winnower. But when the government offered prizes for producing a single harvester that would combine stripping, threshing, winnowing and bagging, Hugh, his father and one of his brothers built a prototype stripper-harvester from bits and pieces of farm machinery. By the early 1890s they'd built an improved model which they marketed as the Sunshine harvester. The Sunshine was an instant success.

Then, when Hugh Victor McKay died in the mid 1920s, he left £2000 to help Flynn's Aerial Medical Service experiment. The bequest was made on the proviso that the Presbyterian Church doubled that amount. The Church okayed the idea and Flynn raised a further £5000. With the money raised, Hudson Fysh honoured his promise of help and Qantas leased to Flynn—on extremely favourable terms—a fabric-covered De Havilland 50 aeroplane, named *Victory*.

On 17 May 1928 *Victory* took off from Cloncurry, Queensland, after the AIM Aerial Medial Service received its first emergency call, no doubt via one of Alf Traeger's famous pedal wirelesses. Arthur Affleck was the pilot and the doctor was St Vincent Welch. And so all the various threads of Flynn's vision of a Flying Doctor Service had now become a reality.

The final part of John Flynn's work began with turning his AIM Aerial Medical Service into a national community service. This vision was far greater than the church could handle by itself. What Flynn now wanted was an arrangement between state and federal governments and the AIM itself. And so the idea of a National Aerial Medical Service of Australia (NAMS) was set into motion. To get it up and running, Flynn travelled throughout Australia addressing public meetings, talking to politicians and holding press interviews until the NAMS became a reality.

The mid 1930s also saw a different role that the two-way radio was to play for the people in remote areas and the children in particular. Around that time John Flynn was looking to establish a base of the Aerial Medical Service in Alice Springs. In doing so he got help from a long-time educationalist named Adelaide Miethke. At that time Miethke was a member of the Council of the Flying Doctor Service of South Australia. And, on a visit to Alice Springs, she saw the potential of the Flying Doctor two-way radio network, not only as a tool for patient–doctor contact and remote community contact but also for educational purposes.

Adelaide Miethke was born in June 1881 at Manoora, South Australia, the sixth daughter of ten children. Her father was a Prussian schoolmaster. She was educated at various country schools and at Woodville Public School before becoming, as had John Flynn, a pupil-teacher. In the early 1900s she attended the University Training College and her first teaching appointment was at Lefevre Peninsula School

A workaholic by nature, by 1915 she was founding president of the Women Teachers' League where she fought to place women as headmistresses. The following year she became the first female vice-president of the South Australian Public School Teachers' Union. She studied part-time to complete her degree and became an Inspector of Schools in late 1924. Miethke applied extremely tough teaching standards. She was a stickler for formality and devoted much of her life to helping improve teachers' industrial conditions and to raising the status of women.

Miethke also believed that 'technically gifted girls should have a chance of developing their bent' and that while 'her home was a woman's place, it need not be her prison'. To that end she also helped set up what were to be known as Central Schools. These were training schools for young women to become housewives of 'skill and taste'. Initially the schools offered pre-vocational training to girls aged thirteen to sixteen. General subjects were studied as well as practical classes in things like laundry work, cookery, household management, first aid, drawing and applied art, needlework and dressmaking. Second-year girls received millinery and secretarial training.

Then after Miethke had become president of the Women's Centenary Council of South Australia, she helped raise money to establish the Alice Springs base of John Flynn's Aerial Medical Service. This was the connection with John Flynn because, by that stage, she'd become the Flying Doctors' state branch's first woman president as well as the editor of the magazine *Air Doctor*. That's when the idea of using the Flying Doctor's two-way radio network to set up a School of the Air came to mind. Some of the teachers at Alice Springs Primary–High School took radio lessons and trials began after a landline was laid from the base to the school. On 8 June 1951 the first broadcasts of School of the Air were made from the Flying Doctor base in Alice Springs.

But, unfortunately, John Flynn didn't get to see the realisation of this part of his grand vision because only a month before School of the Air was officially opened, he died of cancer in Sydney. At his request his ashes were interred at the foot of Mount Gillen, just west of Alice Springs. It was said at his service that: 'Across the lonely places of the land he planted kindness, and from the hearts of those who call those places home, he gathered love'.

In 1955, the designation of 'Royal' was added to the Flying Doctor Service. As was John Flynn's dream, the Royal Flying Doctor Service is a non-profit organisation that provides free health care services to 'all people who live, work or travel in the world's largest medical waiting room'; a waiting room that stretches from Christmas Island in the Indian Ocean to Elizabeth Island in the Great Barrier Reef, and all the states and territories in between.

References:

John Behr, 'Traeger, Alfred Hermann (1895–1980)', *Australian Dictionary of Biography*, Volume 12, Melbourne University Press, 1981, pp. 251–252.

Graeme Bucknall, 'Flynn, John (1880–1951)', *Australian Dictionary of Biography*, Volume 8, Melbourne University Press 1981, pp. 531–534.

Suzanne Edgar and Helen Jones, 'Adelaide Miethke (1881–1962)', *Australian Dictionary of Biography*, Volume 10, Melbourne University Press, 1981, pp. 497–498.

John Lack, 'Hugh Victor McKay (1865–1926)', *Australian Dictionary of Biography*, Volume 10, Melbourne University Press, 1981, pp. 291–294.

J. Percival, 'Fysh, Sir Wilmot Hudson (1895–1974)', *Australian Dictionary of Biography*, Volume 8, Melbourne University Press, 1981, pp. 603–605.

Neil Smith, 'Lt. John Clifford Peel, Australian Flying Corps', essay published online at http://www.3squadron.org.au/subpages/peel.htm.

A Short Little Story

Well, I don't talk too much, so it better be just a short little story. I've lived here in Hungerford, now, for about fifty or sixty years or thereabouts. I guess a lot of people mightn't know where Hungerford is, would they? Well, it's right on the Queensland side of the Dog Fence, between Bourke, in New South Wales, and Thargomindah or, if you go the other way, it's between Bourke and Cunnamulla.

As you can see, there's not too much here other than a few houses, the police station and the pub. I live in one of the houses. But if you go back to the old cemeteries around here and you have a good look at the graves, you'd be lucky to find anyone over fifty. I'd say that most of the graves out there are from around the turn of the century and that's when the big sort of flu epidemic came through. And that killed quite a few people.

Anyhow, not that they were about then, but the Flying Doctor Service flies out here about every month and they have a medical clinic, just to keep a check on us all. They usually come out from Broken Hill, or occasionally from Charleville. They were here just last Thursday, actually. Well, you just ring up and say you want to see the doctor about this or that and so, when they arrive, you join the queue.

Most times it's just the pilot and a doctor or a nurse; then sometimes there's also one woman comes out, what does the women's health.

I've always supported the Flying Doctor. In fact, they started up an annual field day here a few years back and a big part of it was to raise money for the Royal Flying Doctor Service. They did that out here at the sports ground, and that's been going real well; but then they had to put it on every second year so it didn't run into the one that they had in at Broken Hill. And so now Broken Hill has it one year and we have it the next. It's only a one-day turn-out but, oh, they do lots of things, and at the end of the day they have this big auction and all the dealers and wheelers, they put in different things to be sold. Like, someone might hand in a fish or something and, you mightn't believe this, but it might bring in anything between $300 or $400. Yes, just the one fish. No, there was nothing special about it.

About three or four years ago I think it was, they auctioned a rain gauge, and that brought in around $1000. Just between you and me, I don't know why anyone out here would want a rain gauge because it doesn't ever rain that much. It wasn't even raining then. And there was nothing special about that rain gauge, neither. It was just a normal old rain gauge; I'd say, about thirty odd dollars worth in the shop. But, see, what would happen was that one bloke would buy it for, say, $200 or $300, and then he'd donate it back in to the Flying Doctor Service and so then they'd go and put it up for auction again and it'd be sold again for another $150 or $200. And it went along like that till it ended up fetching something like $1000, as I said.

So that was a good little earner for the Flying Doctor.

But living out here like, with the Flying Doctor Service, they can have a plane land in Hungerford within the hour, which is fairly fast. And I've seen quite a few emergencies in my time too, and when they get here they stabilise you first. Sometimes they might bring a paramedic or whatever. Actually, my ex-missus would've been dead if it weren't for the Flying Doctor Service. She was having a heart attack out here some years ago and they were here in around the hour, or a bit over. Sometimes it depends if there's a plane available because they fly thousands of kilometres a year. Yes, it's just unbelievable, isn't it? Anyhow, they flew her down to Broken Hill and I went down in the plane with her. This was about ten years ago now. They had the King Airs back then. But I remember when I first came out here, back in the early 1950s, when they had the de Havilland Dragons. You know, the three-engined thing, with the double wing.

A Team Thing

I've got lots of memories of my time with the Flying Doctor Service but some of it's pretty warped medical humour, really—the type of humour that a lot of readers wouldn't understand. But I think probably the main thing I'd like to say is how it's an incredible team thing, not only with the support staff but also when the doctor, the nurse and the pilot go out.

An example of that would be the time we, unfortunately, bogged the aircraft out at Laura, which is west of Cooktown, on the edge of the Lakefield National Park. I think it might've been the Queen Air or C-90, I'm not exactly sure now, but they had a dirt strip there at Laura and we were flying in for a clinic. So the pilot's coming in to land and there's the local nurse, parked in her car, in a place at the end of the runway, which was making things a bit difficult for our pilot to land. So our pilot's saying, 'What the hell's she parked there for?'

Anyhow, we landed okay and our pilot's taxiing the plane down the strip and he's going on about how dangerous it was for the nurse to park where she had because she could've caused an accident and all that. 'Get outa the bloody way!' he says. Then, after the nurse had moved her car, the pilot went to turn the aeroplane around and he bogged it. So it then became very apparent as to just why the nurse had parked her vehicle over that particular section of the airstrip—to warn him that it was too wet.

Anyhow, we went ahead and we did the clinic that morning. Then once we'd finished the clinic we spent the afternoon digging the aircraft out of the bog. And that turned out to be a real team thing too, because there we all were— the pilot, the doctor and nurse, along with every other able-bodied person in town—all with shovels and so forth, helping get this aeroplane out of the bog.

That's just one incident. Another example was when we had to shut one of the engines down. It was the right-hand engine and because the pilot couldn't leave his seat, he couldn't see out that side of the aeroplane. So he asked me to get up the front, in the cockpit, which I did. Then he got me to look back around the window.

'Can you see the engine?' he asked.

'Yes,' I said.

'Are there any flames?'

Thankfully there weren't.

So not only do we have to work as a team, we've also got to be flexible within that team structure, because there's a lot of times when we might land somewhere and we've got to grab all our gear and get out of the aeroplane and jump into the back of a truck or ute and be driven out along some shockingly rough, slippery, muddy track to where the patient is. And everybody pitches in and helps each other out. Say if there's an accident; usually it's the pilot who's trying to erect a shade the patient or they're standing there holding the IV [intravenous] drip, or maybe the pilot's running backwards and forwards to the aircraft to 'get the big orange pack' or to 'get the little black pack' or whatever, while the doctor and the nurse are busy attending the injured. Naturally we don't overstep our boundaries and we don't cross disciplines but we all help each other out, under direction, and the best we can.

Then there's other times when we've all had to get in a boat and row across a creek to get a patient out of their humpy and bring them back. That actually happened at Bloomfield, which is up in the Daintree National Park. I wasn't the nurse in that case; another nurse was involved. But with that one, it was wet season and this feller was sick and his mate had radioed for help and warned us that the creek was flooded. So the RFDS crew got the message and they flew up there and when they landed they got a lift out to the flooded creek. Then they jumped in a boat and rowed across the creek, and after they got to the other side, they went off to do the house visit. The feller was pretty crook in bed so they then had to get him out of his house, back to the creek, into the boat, then row him back across the flooded creek, where they got a lift back to the airstrip, loaded the patient in the aeroplane, then flew him out to hospital. I mean, that's service, isn't it?

Also, I guess that a lot of the weather-related stories you've heard have been about dust storms and deserts and that. But because Cairns is one of the wettest places in Australia, we get lots of wet ones up here. So getting bogged is probably our worst problem and also not being able to land because of the poor weather or just having to go round and round and round till you just about throw up. And then you have to call it quits because if you did manage to land, you'd get bogged anyway and you wouldn't be able to take off again, and that doesn't help anybody.

Of course, situations like that can be totally devastating, especially if there's an emergency and you can't land the aeroplane. From that point of view, the worst time I remember was when we were running a clinic in Birdsville, which is in the south-western corner of Queensland, just down near the South Australian border. This was back, very early on in the piece, when I was working out of the Charleville base and a lot of the medical calls were still done by radio. Anyway, we got an emergency call through on the radio from a father who lived about 150 miles east of Birdsville. He was in a shed and he was telling us that his son had been electrocuted. But because the airstrip on his property was so wet, unfortunately there was no possible way we could get out there. In fact, it'd been raining so heavily everywhere east of Birdsville that it was heavy flooding. And having to listen to this call on the radio, over the speakers, it was just very, very … well, it stayed with me for a very long time, because basically we were trying to talk the father through CPR (cardiopulmonary resuscitation) and when you're very nervous or upset, like the father was, you get the shakes.

Even medical people sometimes get the shakes in emergency situations. That happens because your body's producing adrenalin in an attempt to try and help you cope with the situation. It's exactly like you've had a big fright or something like that. And when people get like that they think they can feel a pulse when, in reality, they can feel the shaking of their own pulse. And this distraught father thought he could still feel a pulse and he was calling out, 'I can still feel a pulse. I can still feel a pulse' and we were trying to explain that there was no possible way we could get out there and land on his strip because of the flooding. So then he's calling out, 'Quick, get a helicopter then. Quick.'

But it's tough to have to say, 'Sorry, it's just not going to help, because even if we could get a helicopter, it'll be at least eight hours before it reaches you.'

What he didn't understand was that the nearest helicopter would've been at Toowoomba, or maybe even Rockhampton, and even if we could've organised a helicopter, it still would've been five or six hours' flying time away. And there's no way anyone could keep doing CPR for that long and have the person survive. Generally, after thirty minutes that's when you'll make a call. By saying 'make a call', I mean having to make a decision. Usually, if you haven't got any heartbeat back within thirty minutes and you're still doing CPR, well, then you'll 'make a call' and declare the patient dead.

So after being on the radio for at least half an hour and from how the father was describing that his son had turned blue and he was still unresponsive, the doctor was forced to say, 'Look, if you're still having to do CPR and he's not responding, I'm afraid your son's dead.' And the father was still screaming, pleading with us to get a helicopter out there, which, being a parent, you can understand he'd do.

That's probably the saddest story I've got. But we just couldn't get out there because of the wet conditions. Even if it'd been dry it still would've taken, I don't know, maybe an hour or something to fly out there, and that would've also been too late. I mean, we probably would've attempted it because that's the way we are. We never give up. But that was a heartbreaking one that one, was—to hear the father just so, so distressed and there was absolutely nothing we could do about it. Sometimes, logistically, it's a nightmare.

Anyhow, I guess I've got off the track a bit there, because as I said, really the main thing I wanted to get across was that with the doctor, the nurse and the pilot, and even with all the support staff, when you're working for the RFDS, it's an incredible team sort of thing.

Almost but not Quite

I was amazed that in my earlier years as a pilot, with both the Cairns Aerial Ambulance and the Royal Flying Doctor Service, just how we were able to find some of these places, because really we had little to no nav [navigation] aids at all. In fact, I'm certain that somebody up there was looking after us.

Still and all, there were techniques you could use. Like, once you got airborne, if you held the correct heading that you'd flight-planned and you'd allowed for the estimated wind direction and speed, realistically, in the end, you could only be out by as far as the wind forecast was wrong, if you get what I mean. Of course, these weather forecasters, they're human just like the rest of us and while they do their best, at the altitudes we travelled there'd always be the potential for errors in their forecasted winds anyway.

So you'd have to take all that into consideration. For example, if you were flying to a place which is on the coastline say, the Aboriginal Community of Pormpuraaw up in the Gulf, what you'd do was you'd lay off significantly to one side. Then by doing that it'd bring you out five or ten miles north of the community and then, when you came out of the cloud or if it was at night or whatever and you crossed the coast, you knew you had to turn left. But if you didn't allow for that variation and you came across the coast, well, you wouldn't know if you were to the south of Pormpuraaw or the north of Pormpuraaw and you'd then be left with the dilemma of 'which way do I turn?' So those were the sort of techniques we used to use.

But as time went by and we started getting basic navigational aids at some of the remote locations, then you were pretty much home and hosed. By navigational aids I mean things like a non-directional beacon or VHF omniranger. You know, you'd have some sort of electronic guidance to the place via the radio. They call them radio 'nav aids'. Nowadays, of course, a lot of them have been superseded by route navigation based on Global Positioning System (GPS).

In actual fact, I remember the first time we put Global Positioning System in our King Air aircraft. It was after the Gulf War—the first Gulf War, that is—in the early 90s, just when GPS first started becoming available to the aviation community. The end result of this story was actually a bit disappointing but that had nothing to do with the GPS we were trialling. Anyhow, we put a GPS called a Trimble TNL 2000 into our evacuation King Air. There, that's not a bad memory for a bloke who's been out of the game for a fair while, is it? I don't know whether they're still in existence any more, but all of a sudden, with the help of twenty-three satellites or what have you, we were able to go to a geographical point with complete accuracy in all weathers.

Anyhow, a station property along the road up to Musgrave from Laura called us up one afternoon. I think it might've even been Kalinga Station though I'm not a hundred percent sure about that. But it was the middle of the wet season and it was raining and we had a conference here at Cairns that I was involved in. I happened to be on call at the same time so I got dragged away from the conference, with the ever patient nursing sister, and the two of us headed off to this particular property for an 'evac'.

Now, had we not had GPS on board, there was no way in this world—other than by just pure luck—that we would've been able to find the property. But the latitude and longitude of the place were well known and recorded so we were able to enter that into the GPS and it took us straight to the spot.

The only problem was that—and this was the disappointing bit—because it was raining so heavily, visibility was poor. And this is one of the things about visual flying: see, once you come off instrument flying into visual flying, naturally there has to be sufficient visibility for you to conduct a visual approach or what's called a 'circling approach'. That's 'circling', meaning you're making a circuit-type approach rather than straight into a runway. So of course you've got to have sufficient visibility to be able to meet those circling minimum requirements. But on this occasion we didn't have sufficient visibility and each time we tried to make a circuit we'd lose sight of the runway. So it was a case of almost but not quite, and after making three attempts we had to pull out of that one and we never got there.

But, as I said, that had more to do with the prevailing conditions rather than the GPS we were trialling and, as it turned out, three vehicles were already bogged on the airstrip, with the patient, so the odds were that if we'd have landed we wouldn't have been able to help anybody anyway. We'd only have ended up with a stuck aeroplane, which meant that we would've had to tax their fuel by them having to pull us out of the bog, plus taxed their food bill by us having to stay there for a few days until the strip dried out well enough for us to take off again. And so, as I said, all that wouldn't have helped the patient at all.

So, after having found the place with Global Positioning System—and what a tremendous advertisement it was for GPS—we weren't able to finish it off by landing. Anyway, I think it convinced management that the sooner we put GPS into all our aeroplanes the better it'd be for everyone involved. But I must say that it was actually a pretty rare event when a Flying Doctor aeroplane was unable to reach a patient. Anyhow, in the end in that particular case they somehow managed to get a four wheel drive vehicle out to the property and they miraculously evacuated the patient to Laura. Then I think he was brought up by helicopter to Cooktown or something, so it was quite a roundabout route to go. But he did survive.

Are You Sure?

Of course, each and every one of us in the Royal Flying Doctor Service always try to present ourselves to the public in the best light possible. That's a given. It's a simple matter of professionalism.

And, anyway, in the greater scheme of things, this was sort of irrelevant, I guess. But we are talking about 'anecdotal' stories, aren't we? I remember when I was working up in Broken Hill. Back in those days I was the administration officer out at the RFDS Base up there and we had this doctor who used to ride his pushbike out to work, as opposed to drive. It's about a five-or-eight kilometre trip, and it can get very hot in the summer. So he'd just wear any old casual clothes he could find laying around his home, and he'd ride his bike out, knowing that, even if an emergency arose, he always kept a set of nice clean clothes there, out at the base, and all he had to do was have a quick shower, jump into his good clothes, and he'd be ready to fly out in no time flat.

Anyway, he and I were what I'd call mates. You know, he'd always come into my office and we'd have a good chat about this, that and the other. The usual sort of stuff that blokes talk about: the weather and that, mixed with a bit of bull. Then one day he was the doctor-on-call and so in the morning he just threw on some old clothes and he rode out to the base, as per usual. But he'd no sooner got to work than he got paged. It was a priority one. An emergency. I think it was a rollover and there were some fatalities. From memory, it was a family with a caravan, out on the Sydney Road, the other side of either Cobar or Nyngan, somewhere in that area. And with it being a priority like that there's a lot of organising to be done in a very short time. Other than the medical side of things, there's the assessments for a road landing and things like that. Anyhow, all that's okay; everything's ready. He's been given some details—not all, but some, and they're just about ready to go.

The next thing, he comes rushing into my office. 'I've left my clothes at home,' he says. Apparently he'd taken his good clothes home to be washed or something and he'd forgotten to bring them back out to the RFDS Base, as he always did. Well, almost always.

Now, this was back in the good old days when the presentable, and even the fashionable, attire was, you know, the long socks and the good shorts and the open neck shirt. I think it was called the 'Safari era'. So there I was dressed like that and there he was decked out in a dirty old pair of stubby shorts and a tatty old round-neck tee-shirt with, I reckon it might've even been a Newcastle Brown beer logo or something of that description, in the middle of it.

Anyway, as it happened he and I were a similar size and so he looked at me and I looked at him and it was basically, 'No option'. So we disrobed in my office. He takes off his stubbies and tee-shirt. I take off my shorts and shirt and long socks. I think we might've left our footwear as it was. I'm not sure now, but the thing is, I've now got his dirty old stubbies on and his tatty old tee-shirt and he's looking nice and presentable and professional. And so off he flew, out to this high priority along the Broken Hill to Sydney road.

Good, that's all done, and so I go back to work. The next thing, my secretary comes into the office and says, 'There's an official from the Australian Nurses' Federation outside. She's come out to have some discussions with you about our nurses and to see how things are going.'

And there's me, always the one for good presentation and professionalism, and I'm dressed like I've just come in from the garden or somewhere. So this woman comes into the office. She was a good-looking woman; very well presented, very professional looking.

'G'day. I'm John, the admin officer,' I say.

And the shock on her face. You should've seen it. She just stood there, looking me up and down as if to say, 'Are you sure?'

I mean, it was quite embarrassing at the time really, because, as I said, we always try and present ourselves to the public in the best possible light. Still, I guess on that particular occasion, given the circumstances, you could say that I had presented myself in the best available light I could possibly present myself in. But, oh, it was a funny reaction she gave me. I can still remember the look on her face.

Broken

I left school when I was about twelve or thirteen and I got a job out at a place called Ned's Corner Station, which is up there in the top corner of Victoria, New South Wales and South Australia. I'd say that that was in about 1939. So I got this job with a drover, but what I didn't count on was that I'd be working seven days a week for two and sixpence per week. And not only that—I also had to get up and do a two- or two-and-a-half-hour watch every night of the week and live on damper and corned beef; then, for a change, we'd have corned beef and damper.

But anyhow, I stayed with droving for a good long while and over the time I had a few tangles, mainly with horses. Like, four or five years ago I had some special infra-red ray tests on my lungs and they told me that I've had twenty-two broken ribs. Some might be just cracks, I don't know. So you could say that I've not only broken a few horses in, but also a few horses have broken me in too.

There was one time, back when I was pack-horse droving, when a horse kicked my ribs in and I ended up with a big red-blue patch that you could cook a bloody egg on. But anyhow, I kept on working; then ten days later when it was time to come home, I couldn't get up on the horse. So I had to walk all the way back. That one hurt so bad that after a while I went to a doctor and he said that one rib was sitting on top of another and the underneath one was all split. Apparently it'd tried to knit but it kept breaking off and it'd turned into some sort of a big abscess. See, bones have to knit straight; they can't knit crooked. I found that out the hard way.

Then I've also got a few bumps on my foot. See, just there— all those bumps. That happened in '49 or '50 when I broke the bones right across the top, there. It was a Saturday morning, and it'd started to rain, and a couple of mad bullocks had come down from out of the Blue Mountains, so I said, 'I'll just go up and grab these two bullocks.'

So I on the horse flew up a narrow ridge, through wire-grass this high, and the horse went straight into a rabbit warren. He didn't even see the thing. Anyhow, I managed to get clear but when I saw that the horse was trying to get back up, I got back in the saddle. So I got back up but then the horse scrambled in the wet and he slid right down the side of the hill and I went with him.

Now, I don't know exactly what happened but I heard the bones break and I felt my foot crack. I think that the tail of my boot must've hooked against a stone or something and it brought my foot back around like that, twisting it right up, and 'snap'. Then when I looked down, I saw these two bones sticking out of my boot, so I cut the boot off. A good pair of boots, too, they were.

The horse was alright, though. He was better off than me. He was just covered in mud from sliding down the side of the mountain. But then he couldn't get back up to where I was because it was too slippery and there was a fence in his way so I ended up having to crawl for eight hours until I got to help. And I tell you, I was getting a bit worried there for a while because it was still pouring with rain and the gullies were getting fuller and fuller and the water was flowing faster and faster. Anyhow, I eventually made it back.

But a couple of the bones in my foot just wouldn't knit so they had to go and re-break them. That proved to be a bit of a problem too, because it was so hard to get the bones dead straight for them to set and so they had to keep on re-breaking them. In the end I think the foot had to be broken seven or eight times until eventually they set. And then they had to scrape out all the bone chips.

Then there was another droving trip I was on. We hadn't been on the road too long. Anyway, I'd drawn two horses to ride and one of them was pretty flighty, and I knew that if this feller got his head right down he'd do me, so I had to keep his head on his chest. I mean, he was a good horse but he just never wanted to go to work in the morning.

Anyway, one morning just after daylight the bugger threw me and broke my arm. And, oh hell, he done a proper job of it too, because it was all bent around the wrong way. Now this happened somewhere before we got down to Barringun Gate, on the Queensland–New South Wales border. The area was all new to me, but luckily the boss knew his way. So they tucked the arm up there, like that, and they put it in a sling, then the boss and me, we jumped on our horses and off we went for help. Now I reckon we rode for about twenty or thirty mile before we come to a dogger's camp. Doggers are blokes who go out setting dingo traps. Dingoes are a big problem up that way, too. So, anyhow, we got fresh horses there, then we done another twenty mile until we came across a mustering camp. We got fresh horses there again and then we rode another twenty mile to the homestead. I forget the name of the place now, but the Flying Doctor was only an hour or so away and when he come he took me over to the butcher's table.

See, at the homestead there was one of those huge big tables for laying a bullock on to butcher it. The top end was made of wood so that they could cut the beast with knives then the other end was steel so that you could slide half a bullock around. I mean, it was a pretty solid table, bolted down to the floor and all. And it had to be, because you didn't want it to tip over when you dumped a bullock on it. But anyhow, running at an angle from the table to just down the legs, there were these iron stays. Now as I said, my arm was pretty badly broken and for it to have any chance to set, first they had to straighten it out. So they just put my broken arm through one of these stays and the doctor got his feet against the table and he yanked like hell on the arm until he got it back into position. Boy, it hurt. I reckon my eyes just about shot off in different directions, all at the same time.

'There you go,' the doctor said. 'That didn't hurt much, did it?'

Like bloody hell. I mean, it was my arm that was broke, not bloody his.

Anyhow, after the Flying Doctor bloke pulled my arm back together, he plastered it up and I went out and I sat in the sun to let it dry off a bit. Then at about five o'clock that night, after I'd had a cup of tea and a bite to eat, the boss and me, we set out again and we relayed horses all the way back until we got to our camp at daylight, just in time for me to start work again. Anyhow, with my broken arm all plastered up, I picked out a nice quiet horse this time.

But I tell you, that night I was never so pleased to see a dinner camp in my life. Then one of the other blokes, a ringer mate of mine, a blackfella, he said, 'Don't worry, Dusty, I'll do yer watch tonight. She'll be alright.'

'Beaut,' I said, and I didn't even wait to have dinner. I just went and curled up in my swag and I slept for hours.

Then about six weeks later I was supposed to go back to the Flying Doctor to get the plaster cut off. But I didn't bother about that. 'Blow it,' I said, and I just got a pair of tin snips and I cut the bugger off myself.

Burns

I worked as a doctor for the Royal Flying Doctor Service for fifteen years and, while it was a very rich and rewarding experience, oh, we had some very harrowing things to deal with. Because unfortunately not all our retrievals lead to happy endings. But if you've got a job to do, you just do it and that's all there is about it. That's the doctor's edict, isn't it? But in my experience, extremely severe burns cases are probably the hardest ones to deal with, because if the veins have been burnt then you can't get the cannula in, to give them fluids—and they need lots of fluids—plus, of course, there's the intravenous analgesics to relieve the pain.

For example, I got a call once on the HF radio that a fellow had gone out on his motorbike to burn off windrows of scrub on his station property. He was by himself and he had some sort of fire lighting machine, or flame thrower, tied around his neck, which ran on a combination of diesel and petrol. So he was lighting the windrows of scrub with this machine and whether he had the wrong fuel combination in it or what I don't know, but, anyway it exploded while it was still attached to his neck and he received full thickness burns and partial thickness burns to over fifty percent of his entire body surface area.

As I said, this fellow was by himself. What's more, he had no means of communication with his home base. So he rolled on the ground to put the flames out then, with these extensive burns to his body, he got on his motorbike and he rode eighteen kilometres back to his home, opening and closing three gates along the way. And that was an amazing act. Because you know how in the bush it's continually drummed into us to 'always leave the gates as you find them.' Of course, you wouldn't expect someone to follow that rule when they have fifty percent body surface area burns, would you? But he did. This fellow, he did it to a tee. He opened and closed three gates along the eighteen-kilometre journey back to get help. So it's really ingrained in people, isn't it—'always leave gates as you find them.'

Anyway, he finally arrived at the homestead and that's when we got the call. So the pilot flew the nurse and I out there where, first of all, we resuscitated him. Then we prepared him for transport by putting in an indwelling catheter to catch his urine. We then loaded him in the plane and headed off to the Royal Brisbane Hospital. And this fellow was in such a bad way that on the flight down to Brisbane his urine was just solid myogliomicurea, from the muscle which had been burnt. So you could say that he was sort of urinating melted muscle.

But he died, the poor fellow, four or five days later on, in the Burns Unit at the Royal Brisbane Hospital. But, once again, as distressing as it was, that was a story of just sheer courage in my books. 'Always leave gates as you find them.'

Another extremely distressing event was when we got a call that two fellows had been burnt in an explosion at an oil rig, out on the South Australian border. The most serious of the two had received burns to over ninety percent of his body surface area. He was still alive but he'd inhaled the flames, which meant that he'd burnt his lungs as well.

Now, the second fellow, the one with the least burns, he pulled through eventually so I'll concentrate on the problems we had with the most seriously burnt fellow. When we got out there, firstly I had to try and find a vein where there were no burns. With having burns to over ninety percent of his body, that was difficult. In the end, the only place I could cannulate him was down at his ankle. I then put him to sleep—paralysed him—then I had to put an intratracheal tube into his trachea so that I could ventilate him. This also caused problems as his vocal cords had also been partially burnt and I had to split them before I could get the intratracheal tube into him. I was then faced with a greater problem; perhaps a more ethical one. I had a pretty fair idea that this fellow was going to die. But, if at all possible, I wanted him to remain alive at least until his relatives could see him before he did die. And as our destination was the Royal Brisbane Hospital, that meant we'd have to keep him going for a fair number of hours. So we loaded the two fellows into the aeroplane and we called up another RFDS plane and we organised to meet halfway, at Charleville.

At Charleville we performed an escharotomy on the most serious of the two fellows, which entailed the cutting of burnt tissue. See, skin tissue, when it burns, contracts and causes a blockage of the blood flow, which doesn't allow the chest to expand for respiration purposes. So we did an escharotomy on him at Charleville and then we put him in the other plane and they took him down to Brisbane.

And that was that. His family did get to see him while he was still alive. Whether they wanted to or not, I don't know, because he was just a black, black charred mess. But it was very horrible from my point of view having to do these things, and it was also an extremely exhausting and emotional time, because the poor fellow of course died, as I figured he would.

Call the Doctor!

By the late 1970s, early '80s, we'd well and truly established our station property, which was about 350 kilometres out from Kalgoorlie, in Western Australia. I was managing the place by this stage and one year we had a team of shearers from New Zealand come through, a large number of whom were Maoris. Anyhow, one morning one of the Maori chaps was shearing away and his handpiece jammed and it flew around and cut him severely on the forearm. With blood gushing everywhere, the first thing his mates did was to grab a towel and wrap it around his arm in an attempt to stem the flow. But this was only a temporary measure because it was obvious that urgent medical help was required.

At the time of the accident, I was working out in the sheep yards and the first thing that I knew about it was when one of the shearers came rushing out from the shed. 'There's been a serious accident,' he called. 'Is there any way we can get in touch with a doctor, and fast?'

Now, I'll just remind you that we were 350 kilometres or so from the nearest hospital. But, as luck would have it, I had the portable radio in the car. So I got straight onto the Flying Doctor base in Kalgoorlie and told them about the problem and how the shearer was in dire need of help.

'Well actually,' the person at the base said, 'at this moment there's a plane on its way back to Kalgoorlie from a clinic run out along the Eyre Highway and Trans-line. We'll divert them. And don't worry,' the person added, 'they should be there in a few minutes.'

So I raced the four kilometres or so down to the homestead then I drove on down to the airstrip. The plane arrived not long after and I rushed the doctor back up to the wool shed, where he got straight in and treated the injured shearer.

Now, in this particular case the doctor had arrived on the scene of the accident within an hour. So you can imagine what this team of New Zealand shearers was thinking. They couldn't believe it. Here was one of their mates, having been severely injured, right out on the Nullarbor, which is out in the middle of nowhere, hundreds of kilometres from the nearest town, and help arrived so quickly. Within the hour. To them, it was almost unbelievable, and of course, it brought home the huge importance of the Royal Flying Doctor Service, not only for the shearers themselves but they also realised just how important the RFDS is to everyone living out in these remote areas.

And so appreciative of the service were these New Zealand shearers that, at the end of the shearing they decided to donate an hour's time in aid of the RFDS. That is, each of the shearers gave one hour's shearing time, the shed hands gave one hour's wages; everyone did, right through to the contractor himself. And for what was an eight-stand team, this ended up making quite a sizable cheque. Then, when the next-door neighbour heard about this, he also cottoned on to the idea. Better still, he had a bigger flock and a bigger shed and of course a bigger team, which in turn translated into an even bigger cheque.

In the end, this giving of time became an annual fundraising event throughout the area. As a follow-on from that, all the shearing contractors in Western Australia ended up establishing a state-wide appeal, with the shearers and such donating an hour of their working time and with all the proceeds going to the RFDS.

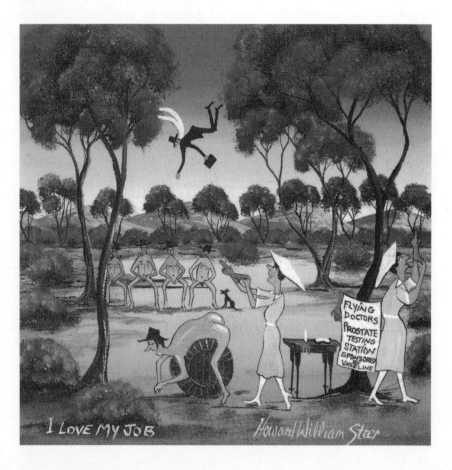

Camp Pie

I first started with the RFDS as a flight nurse up in Port Augusta, South Australia, then I went down to Adelaide for a while and now this is my third year up in the Northern Territory, working out of Alice Springs. Initially, I used to get terribly airsick. Oh, for the first three weeks I remember I was as sick as a dog. Then one day I just suddenly got over it, thank goodness, and now I don't have a problem with airsickness, not even when we're going through the roughest of conditions.

Actually, I remember when the turn-about took place. We were flying a young guy back after he'd somehow been blown out of a cherry-picker and had broken just about every bone in his body. This was before we had pressurised aircraft so we had to fly at around the 2000-feet level. I knew it was going to be rough so as we were about to take off my first thought was, 'Here we go again. I'm going to be airsick.'

Anyhow, we took off and as we were flying along, getting bounced around, the doctor wasn't offering a great deal of help and so all of my focus was on this seriously injured patient. Then when I turned around to ask the doctor if he might lend me a hand, there he was with his head stuck in a sick bag, really going for it. Great help, ay. And at that exact moment it struck me: 'Hey, I don't get airsick any more.' And I haven't been airsick since.

But some people just really struggle to adjust to working inside an aircraft while it's in flight. Another time, I remember, we had a paediatrician out with us—he was only a new chap—and we flew from Port Augusta, out to Cooper Pedy, on to Yalata, then back to Port Augusta, and he threw up all the way. Mind you, at the time I was pretty annoyed with him. But then after a while you look back on those sort of things as humorous events, don't you?

One that wasn't so funny was when I first came up here to Alice Springs and we flew out to a community in the Pitjantjatjara Lands for a guy who'd had a heart attack. By the time we arrived it was dark and, so that we could land, the pilot had to activate the lighting on the strip. Then when we walked into the emergency room, this crook bloke, he was very, very sick indeed. Actually, he was grey. After doing ECGs, we decided that we had to give him a couple of doses of a certain medication that helps dissolve the clots in the heart.

Then, just as we were giving him the first dose, a huge thunderstorm hit. Absolutely huge it was, and the lightning struck the power supply and all the lights went out in the community. So we didn't have any lights. Anyhow, the second dose of the medication had to be given thirty minutes after the first dose, that's providing no abnormalities develop in the patient's heart reading. At that stage we were monitoring him with a torch, on the life pack, in an attempt to gauge whether to give him this second dose or not.

In the meantime our pilot's out at the generator, with the essential services officer, trying to see if they can fix the power because the doctor was keen to fax off copies of the ECG to the specialist in Alice Springs. And of course without power, the fax machine wasn't working. The phones weren't working either and we also needed power to light the airstrip so that we could take off. So we waited for half an hour and in the end we just decided to go ahead and give the second dose by torchlight. Then, just as we were doing that, the ambulance drove up and its lights shone straight into the emergency room and we discovered, 'Oh, we've now got light.' So we did the rest by the headlights of the ambulance, and everything went beautifully.

Anyhow, we finished the treatment and we gave the patient pain relief. Finally they got the power back on and the lights sorted out so we prepared the patient and we headed out to the airstrip. Then just as we started getting ready to load the stretcher, the heavens opened again and it just bucketed down. Absolutely bucketed down. There was water everywhere. The only person that was dry was the patient because we'd put a plastic sheet over him.

Of course, now the pilot's on edge because a heavy downpour on a dirt strip can make for an extremely difficult take-off. What's more, the plane was a Pilatus PC-12, which is worth something like five or six million dollars, all decked out. They're like a flying hospital. Basically, they've got everything you'd need in an ICU Unit. So they're very expensive things, which was why the pilot was so on edge. The last thing he'd want to do was to drop the thing or bog it or damage it in any way.

Anyhow, there we were, soaked to the bone and freezing cold. Still, we managed to get the patient into the plane and after a careful assessment we took of. But because of the thunderstorm, it was an extremely rough flight and by now I'm going through the possibilities of 'What else could go wrong'. So I made the patient as comfortable as I could and made doubly sure that everything was nice and tight and secure.

'Good,' I said to myself, 'now I can relax a bit.'

No sooner had I said that than the patient started vomiting. And that was the final straw because now there were bits of camp pie being sprayed all over the place. Anyway, we eventually landed back in Alice Springs. The storm was over by then and the next day they flew the patient down to Adelaide, where he had bypass surgery. So it all worked out well for him. But we were left to clean his mess out of the plane and then, of course, my uniform also had chuck all through it. It was just shocking. There was camp pie everywhere.

Captain 'Norty'

Because my name's Norton Gill, everyone out at the base knows me as 'Capt Norty'. So you could say that my wife has a 'Norty' in bed with her every night. I've been a pilot with the RFDS for twenty-four years or so now. And, yes, I still enjoy it. When I get that call at two o'clock in the morning or whenever, I still get out of bed and I just go out there and I do it. But I'm going on sixty years old and I've only got a year and a bit to go before I retire. And when that happens, my wife, Margaret, and I, we'll join the grey nomads and drive around Australia.

But oh, sometimes these aeroplanes can play tricks and, you know, when they do they can really put the wind up you. I can remember going from Cairns over to the Gulf of Carpentaria one time to visit the Kowanyama Aboriginal Community. I was flying a King Air that had just come out of maintenance. Anyhow, it was coming on dark so the sun was just going down. I had the doctor sitting up front with me—a bloke called Gary—when all of a sudden an alarm came on to say that we had a fire in the left-hand side motor or, in flying terms, the port motor.

'What's that?' Gary called out.

'It's the fire alarm,' I said.

Well, he mustn't have comprehended that straight away because he said, 'What, have we got a fire?'

So I had a bit of a look out of my side window and I said, 'No, I don't think so. I can't see anything.'

And that's what you do. If you get a fire warning in these aeroplanes, the first thing you do is have a look and see if there's any smoke coming out anywhere. Then if there is, the first thing you do is close down the motor. It's not really such a big drama. I mean, you've got systems in place. There's fire extinguishers on board and all that to put a fire out. But I've never heard of one ever catching fire.

But the thing that did concern me was that if this King Air had just come out of maintenance, well, it does make you wonder, doesn't it? Anyhow, we continued flying along with Gary, the doctor, breaking out into a sweat while he's sniffing here and there, just in case he can detect smoke. Then, would you believe it, a couple of seconds later the right-hand, or starboard, motor fire alarm comes on. So then we had two fire alarms going. And if poor old Gary wasn't pretty twitchy beforehand, he certainly was now.

'Is there another fire?' he asked.

'Well,' I said, 'look out your side window. Can you see any smoke?'

So he craned his neck as far as it could go. 'No, I don't think so,' he said.

'Well,' I said, 'just you watch this,' and I turned the aircraft about forty-five degrees and, when I did, both the fire alarms went out, just like that. So then he started to relax … just a tiny bit.

But see, what happened in those older model King Airs was that if the sun was at just the right angle it shone, or reflected, through a small gap somewhere and it used to hit these little sensor things inside the motor. That's when you'd get the fire alarm coming on. I mean, you didn't even need sunlight. The same thing used to happen back when I was doing night freight and sometimes you'd start up under normal electric light and a fire alarm would come on. Then, very occasionally, they'd even come on in the rain.

Anyhow, it was quite an interesting thing to have both alarms come on. That was extremely unusual. But it wasn't fire. And in those King Airs they had a turbine motor—the Pratt and Whitney PT-6s—and really I've never heard of any of them ever catching fire. It was just that they had these old fire sensors in them, that's all. So yes, poor old Gary, he got quite twitchy about it all. It really put the wind up him. Mind you, I must admit it initially put the wind up me too, especially when both the port and starboard fire alarms came on.

Coen

Yes, well, my husband Col and I weren't rich or anything. We were country people so we just 'made do', if you know what I mean. Anyhow, when Col finished up bee farming— he was a honey man—he wanted to go and see his sister, Jess, who was working up at Coen, almost to the top of Cape York Peninsula in Queensland. After Col retired we still had his work truck so we took the wheels off a little old caravan and we bolted the caravan onto the back of the truck and we went all the way up in that to see Jess. And, oh, what a journey it was. There were times when I was afraid we'd never get home.

Jess was nursing at the Australian Inland Mission Hospital up there. At that time, the last three tribes of full-blood black Aborigines were also living there. The mission had a hostel for them so that they could have their children taught. But, oh, it was very, very primitive. There was no electricity. They did have generators but they didn't run all the time. Then the phone—you could only use it at certain hours; like you could only get through in the evening or something like that.

But Jess had been thoroughly trained in nursing. In her early days she'd been a Bush Nurse and she'd go around on horseback. She could do anything, just about. And she had to up there too, because there was no doctor up in Coen. The nurse had to do everything. She was three years up there, and that was at the end of her nursing because she was an older woman by then. Her sight was going and she could only manage to do so much for so long.

From memory, the main part of the mission at Coen was all combined in the one building. Then, as far as white people went, there was a lady and her husband running the hostel part. The man was a lay preacher and his wife did the cooking and looked after the children in the hostel part. Jess had a portion of that building as her clinic, and it was a nursing home as well. Now, I don't know how many years the lay preacher and his wife had been working there. I suppose they could've stayed for as long as they wanted to actually, because not too many people would want to go up and live in a place like that.

Now, I'm not exactly sure what the Aboriginal people did because most of them were quite old. The older ones were kept in a separate part. They were living in either brick or cement buildings, which were quite basic. You know, just sort of a building with a room and a stove and a bed. It was just simple. And the government supplied everything for those Aboriginal tribes because they were very primitive and they had all their dogs. They were still walking around with bare feet and they hardly wore any clothes. Really, to be honest, they much preferred to live outside and have a little tiny fire on the ground, like they did in their natural way—like they were used to doing.

With any of the more serious medical problems or injuries, Jess would have to get on the radio and ask the Flying Doctor Service to come up and fly the patients back down to Cairns. Oh, and, of course, she was very well trained as a midwife. So yes, Jess did it all, she even sewed up their wounds, because the Aborigines were on welfare and they were allowed to drink and so there was always trouble. Jess not only had to nurse them, she also had to go around each day and she'd have all their medications ready and everything.

But she did have one couple there, with a little boy, and they were described as Islanders. They weren't the full-blood Aborigines like the three remnant tribes were. I met them and Col and I were taken to where they lived, and they were different altogether because they had a garden and they knew how to farm and grow things like fruit trees and all that.

Then, for the younger black women who had husbands and children, the government had built them cottages. These cottages were designed like our normal houses, but they were all aluminium—the walls, the roof, everything. And the government sent up a lady to supervise that section of it and to keep an eye on things. Anyway, this supervisor lady turned out to be good company for Jess because she helped Jess supervise the young women and their husbands and their children and their babies.

Anyhow, it took Col and I ten days to get from Gosford up to Coen. Also the truck was quite old and so Col didn't want to rush. Well, he couldn't rush really. It was a diesel and you didn't rush diesels in those days. But I tell you, the roads, well, they'd get washed away in the wet season, then they'd fix them up again and they'd get washed away again, and all the crossings were washed away. It was shocking. Luckily we didn't travel in the summer. I think it might've even been autumn. The weather was pretty reasonable anyway, because the creeks were quite dry, though you had to be very careful when you were crossing them, with all the sharp rocks and everything.

I mean, well Col's a bushman but just the same, he wasn't a bushman for that sort of country. So it was a real struggle to get up there and we did break down a couple of times. The first time, luckily a man came along with his big truck, which was loaded with supplies for the shop in Coen, and he said, 'For heaven's sake, come behind me or you'll never get there.' So that's how we came to travel behind him, and we felt a bit safer then.

Then, when we finally made it to Coen, we broke down again and they said, 'Well, we'll have to send to the coast for the part,' and when the part didn't arrive when it was supposed to they said, 'You're in Queensland now, so you'll have to wait until the next load comes because they forgot to put it on the truck.' As I said, that was a long time ago now and so I suppose things would've changed a bit in Queensland by now. I hope so anyway.

But of course my big worry was, 'How on earth are we going to get back home?' I thought we'd be stuck there forever because by that stage the tyres on Col's truck were badly worn and we had to go back through crossings that were full of sharp rocks and logs and things. It was just terrible. It just wasn't suitable for tourists.

But then, coming back from Coen, we hardly had any trouble at all. See, it's when you go out into the unknown, into somewhere different like that, that's when you have all the worries. But once you've done it, then the fear's gone.

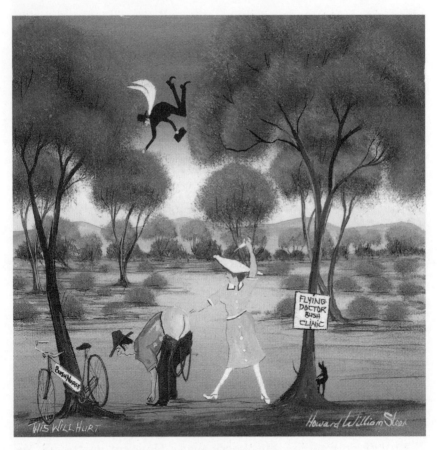

Dad

I'm sure you've heard the term 'mantle of safety'. That encapsulated John Flynn's dream to cover all aspects of care for those who lived and worked in the outback. So, with Flynn as its driving force, the Australian Inland Mission set up hospitals and sent trained nurses out to those remote areas. Then the Flying Doctor Service more or less supported the services of the AIM, plus the many other outback support organisations.

Another important part of Flynn's 'mantle of safety' was to also provide spiritual care and it was to that end that my father, Fred McKay, was recruited by Flynn in 1936 to go out in his International truck and work as a patrol padre, throughout western Queensland. Now these patrol padres were never heavily evangelical or anything. They tended to be more of a comforting presence to people. I mean, yes, they did weddings. They did baptisms. They did burials. They did all those sorts of things. But they were especially trained to meet outback people on their own level. As Dad used to say, 'I meet people where their greatest need is.' So being the pretty handy sort of fellow he was, Dad was always willing to hop in and work in a stockyard or he'd help out doing odd jobs around station homesteads.

Of course, having such a vast area to cover, the truck—the International—was really his home and Dad would sleep out by himself a lot of the time. So the funny thing was that when Dad and Mum married in 1938 and planned to travel together, Mum's parents were so alarmed at what they thought their daughter was getting herself in for, they made sure that Mum at least had something to sleep in, so they bought her a swag. In fact, the bulk of their wedding presents consisted of camping equipment; things like billy cans and tin plates and all that.

Also, by then, Alf Traeger had come up with his pedal-driven radio and for a lot of that earlier time Dad's only communication with the outside world was via the Traeger pedal radio. Really, the pedal radio was the link between the outback people, the Flying Doctor, the AIM hospitals, the patrol padres and the other care organisations who had set up missions out in different places as well.

So Dad carried the pedal radio around in the truck and maintained very close contact and ties with the various Flying Doctor bases and so forth. And perhaps I mightn't even be here today if it wasn't for the pedal radio. Because it was in about November 1938, when my mother was pregnant with me, that they were travelling out in south-western Queensland and they broke a king pin in the truck. It was one of those things that Dad had been assured would never happen to an International truck. But it did. And I've still got the broken king pin. It sits in our lounge room. Anyhow, the king pin broke and of course one wheel collapsed. I mean,

Dad was a pretty good mechanic and he could do most running repairs but he certainly wasn't able to do anything as major as that. It was a crucial piece of equipment and couldn't be replaced, and certainly not out there.

So Dad and Mum found themselves stuck in a claypan near a place called Cuddapan which was about fifty kilometres, in a direct line, from Tanbar Station. You wouldn't find Cuddapan on a map these days but the closest large place was Windorah, which was about 110 kilometres further on from where they broke down. Anyway, there they were— stuck—and so Dad got on his pedal radio and sent out the message. Then after he'd sent the message he walked back along the track, leaving Mum in the truck. So there was my mother, pregnant with me and worried if she'd ever see Dad again and even whether she was ever going to get out of the situation alive. Anyhow, the fellow from Tanbar Station heard the message. Luckily he knew the area quite well so he drove out and he met up with Dad and then they came back and pulled the International out of the claypan, much to Mum's relief.

That's the story I grew up with anyway. But as to other stories, you know, there were stories of Dad's patrol days; stories told by some of these hard-bitten bushmen in the early days of the Flying Doctor Service. One I remember was about an Aboriginal stockman who'd been out mustering and was seriously injured after being thrown from his horse. As luck would have it, Dad was visiting the stockmen's camp on his way through so he threw his aerial up in a tree and got on the radio and called the nearest Flying Doctor base, then he stayed there with the mustering crew until the plane arrived. But of course back in those early days, finding somewhere for the plane to land in many of those remote outback places was a bit of a dicey business too and they often had to chop down scrub to clear a makeshift airstrip. Actually, sometimes it was a bit of a miracle when they did ever somehow land and then take off again.

Anyway, so they cleared a bit of a space and the Flying Doctor's plane landed safely and they picked up this injured Aboriginal stockman. Then, as the plane took off into the sky, one of the old blokes in the camp looked up and when he saw that the shape of the aeroplane, with its wings and body, resembled a cross in the sky, he said to Dad, 'Well, if that isn't the flying Christ, Padre, I don't know what is.'

So that's just another small story. But really, I guess we, as a family, have learned a lot more about our parents and their early years from reading their diaries rather than hearing a lot of stories. I mean, we used to hear Dad telling other people's stories but they were probably very much embellished and some of them, I recall, were unprintable. But their diaries were different because I think, in retrospect, some of the things they wrote then are more meaningful to me now. There was of course lots about everyday, normal things but then there were the hardships of travelling around the bush in a truck. There were the terrible roads, the extremes of the heat, cold and rain, plus there were all the unexpected events, both good and bad. Then of course there were times of great loneliness, when Dad was out there by himself or, later on, when it was just the two of them.

Though the thing that's most important to me is to read of the sacrifices they made in just trying to be there for other people and it was those sacrifices that made them both realise just why they were meant to be there. Even after Dad died, time and time again it was an absolute revelation to us as a family to read or hear about just how much of a part he'd played in the lives of so many many Australians.

But that was Dad's life's work. Even right up until his last years, when he was in his eighties, people would always be asking him to do something or other and no matter how tired or busy he was he'd always help them out in whatever way he could. Then, when we'd ask him why he continued to work so hard, he'd say, 'Well, it's my calling. This is what I'm meant to be doing. This is why I'm here.'

Difficult Conditions

When I was flying for the RFDS, as far as difficult conditions went, the weather was always the telling factor. It still probably is, though nowadays the aeroplanes are far better equipped to handle most things. I mean, we never had any of these modern 'nav' aids or anything so we just had to do the best we could. But things could became scary at times. Thunderstorms are usually the most dangerous, mainly because of the turbulence. To blunder into one of those is not such a good thing. If you try to pull your plane out of the thunderstorm there's the chance that you might rip the wings off and then you end up with a wreckage trail of over five kilometres. I saw just recently up in New South Wales, a plane was torn to pieces in a thunderstorm. So anyone who reckons that thunderstorms aren't scary, well, I'd say they're telling fibs.

Also, up in the higher levels, along with the turbulence you can get hail and that can do terrific damage. Big hail stones can wreck an aeroplane by damaging the front or battering the wings. But of course these days they've got radar and that can pick up the solids that are associated with a thunderstorm, like rain and the hail. And you also have what's called storm-scopes. They can detect the electrical discharge, which gives you a much more accurate picture. Storm-scopes also come in handy when you hit dry thunderstorms. A dry thunderstorm's one that's got no hail or rain in it. Some of them have lightning but mainly it's just severe turbulence. So if you hit a dry thunderstorm, all you can do is to try and hang on until you get spat out the other side of it.

Other than the thunderstorms, there's dust storms. I remember once flying a Navajo out to a station property on the Nullarbor, north of Tarcoola. Someone had had an accident on a motorbike and they needed to be picked up. But on our way out we got stuck in the middle of this hell of a dust storm. And, try as I might, I just could not see a bloody thing. In fact, I never actually found the property that we were supposed to be going out to and in the end I even had quite a job finding my way back home to Port Augusta. That's how crook it was, and rough too.

Fog's another difficulty that we were likely to face. I remember when a call came through that a crop sprayer had had a plane prang down at Naracoorte, in the south-east of South Australia. He happened to be a very good friend of mine, actually. He's okay now, but he was spraying and he flew straight into this great gum tree. Anyhow, we got there at night and there was this fog. Real thick stuff, it was. Now, Naracoorte's notoriously bad for fog, especially at night. So we sort of pushed the limits a bit and we landed in this blooming fog, which would be a definite big 'no-no' these days. You just don't do stuff like that now because of all the rules and regulations they've got in place. But that was a pretty dangerous flight.

So then, let me think: what other sort of difficult conditions were we likely to face? Well, there'd be dirt airstrips, especially after rain. You know, it's as wet as a shag, you land your plane and you get bogged. And believe me, aeroplanes are very easy things to bog and they're terribly hard things to get out once you've bogged them. Usually, before we flew out anywhere we'd check the conditions with the station owners or communities and if there was any doubt at all we'd ask them to go out and drive up and down the strip to see if it was firm enough for the plane to land. If their vehicle left wheel tracks, it was a sign that you could well end up in trouble. Also, of course, by asking them to do that, you'd have to rely on their judgement and most times they'd bias the safety aspect their way and not yours because, especially in an emergency, they'd just be so desperate to get you out there.

As well as that, depending on where you were going, you could ask them to do a run along the airstrip to clear any stock that might be wandering around the place. Then there's always the ongoing problem of the native wildlife like the emus and the roos. You can't do much about them because they'd come out of nowhere and just jump in front of you. And a roo, in particular, can do a terrific amount of damage, because if they hit right on the nose bill, the nose bill could collapse.

Actually, I was pretty lucky with the emus and the roos really, because most of the ones I hit ran through the prop, which basically just chopped them up. I remember at Port

Augusta when the RFDS was thinking about buying the Pilatus PC 12 aeroplanes and we had all these guys coming out from Switzerland, picking our brains as to what sort of conditions we were operating in. Basically they were pretty keen to get it right, which they did.

Anyway, this particular time we had a salesman from Pilatus with us and this guy had no idea as to what outback Australia was like and what sort of conditions the Pilatus aeroplane would have to operate in. So we took him for a trip in the King Air, over the Flinders Ranges to Marree then to Nepabunna Aboriginal Community. Nepabunna was a bit of a doozey, actually. It's stuck right in a valley, with high hills all around, and you had to approach it and take off in the one direction—it's what's called a 'one-way strip'—and so we needed a plane with a good climb rate. So we landed there, at Nepabunna, and Nepabunna was a typical example of a stony airstrip. And this guy from Pilatus, well, he'd never seen anything like it. He was so impressed that he even took a handful of stones back to Switzerland to show them just what we were landing on.

I wasn't actually the pilot that time, so when it came time to leave Nepabunna I was sitting in the back and we were just taking off and the next thing, 'Bang!' There's this terrific jolt as we hit this bloody kangaroo fair in the right-hand propeller and we chewed him up into little pieces. Anyhow, we inspected the prop and one blade had a bit of a woof in it. Still, it didn't look too bad so we decided to take off anyway. It wasn't my decision because I wasn't the pilot but you could feel the vibration through the aeroplane as we were flying along. It shook us around a bit. Of course, once again you wouldn't do that these days—you know, take off after an accident like that. That sort of stuff just doesn't go on now.

Then I guess another difficulty we had, especially in the early days, was the night landings. Before we started using flares we used to use cars to light up the strip at night. One time I remember, up at Marla Bore, in the far north of South Australia; this was back when there was only a roadhouse at Marla and it was virtually just about an all-dirt road right the way from Port Augusta up to Alice Springs. Anyhow, this truck missed a by-pass around some wet ground and it rolled over with two blokes in it. It was a terrible accident. One of the drivers was crushed in the cabin and it took ages to get the other feller out of the wreck.

But, as I said, they weren't using flares in those days so a heap of vehicles went out and parked each side of the runway, and they sat there with their headlights on so that we could see where to land. The only trouble was that they sort of misjudged it a bit and when we landed there was only a whisker in between our wings and their bull bars. So after a few experiences like that, it then became a gradual process to educate settlements and communities into having night flares. And eventually everyone got those, which saved that mad scramble of trying to get as many cars as you possibly could to come and line up along the airstrip in the dark.

With the flares, the basic ones were either kerosene or diesel in a tin or the battery operated ones. Batteries were a bit of a problem because if you don't use them for a few months the batteries can go flat. Plus, batteries are very expensive. So really, the mix of diesel and sand proved the best. They were cheap and quick and easy to organise because the station people usually had all that stuff lying around the place anyway. You just grab a can or a milk tin or an old oil tin, fill it with sand, stick some rag in it, then you soak the sand with diesel, throw in a match and you've got a good flare that will last a fair while—cheap and easy. What's more, on a good night you could see them from about thirty miles away, no worries. Of course, if somebody mistakenly put in a bit too much diesel they could set fire to the countryside and then you'd get your direction from a hell of a lot further away than thirty miles.

So yes, I guess that's a few of the difficulties us pilots could face. But as the years go by you tend to pick up on what's good and what's bad and so your judgement becomes a little better. Experience has a lot to do with it because you can't be taught about a lot of things. Only experience teaches you.

But one last story—one with a little bit of humour to it— and this has to do with turbulence. I was still at Port Augusta back then and there was this big meeting happening up at Mount Willoughby or one of those places up that way. So there were quite a few 'bigwigs', as I'll call them for the sake of the story, who needed to be flown up to this meeting. I was in the King Air and just as we were on descent into Mount Willoughby we suddenly hit severe turbulence. And as we were going through this turbulence, I heard this sort of commotion going on from down the back of the plane. So I took a quick glance around and, for the life of me, I thought I saw this bloody possum running down the aisle. Then, in the split second while I was trying to work out how on earth a possum had got on board, this woman came chasing after it and she grabbed it in a flash and then she stuck it back on her head. That's what I meant by 'bigwig', and even when we landed it still looked a bit skew-whiff to me. I tell you, I wasn't the only one who was trying very hard not to laugh.

Disappearing Flares

This was an interesting one. It was actually with the same doctor, Gary, I'd put the wind up on a previous occasion when he thought we were about to go up in flames midair. So even before we took off, Gary seemed a bit jittery. We were going up to Cape Flattery. Cape Flattery's a mining place, on the eastern side of Cape York Peninsula north of Cooktown, not far from Lizard Island. It's still operational today as a sand and silicon mine. I think Mitsubishi is the crowd that operates it.

Anyhow, one night we got a call to go up there to Cape Flattery to pick up a lady who was reported to be swimming straight out to sea. And because it's full of crocodiles the local people were naturally getting a bit concerned about her welfare and so for her own safety they wanted her out of the place. Really, I think that basically she was a bit funny in the head, because apparently it was a yearly thing she did in an attempt to try and get the RFDS to give her a free trip down to Cairns 'to do a bit of shopping'.

To explain what I mean by 'to do a bit of shopping' ... Well, I often think a lot of these people are a lot smarter than you and me. So they throw a bit of a 'wobbly' and do something strange or mad, which puts the wind up everyone, and so the community wants them out of the place. Basically, it's all a set-up really. Of course, we don't charge any of our patients so they end up getting a free flight to town. Then after they arrive in Cairns they're taken to hospital where they're fed and watered for a day or two. Then they're released from hospital and away they go, 'off to do some shopping', you see. Well, that's just my take on it, of course.

But anyway, so it's night time and the chap who normally put the flares out for us at Cape Flattery wasn't there on this particular occasion. He was away somewhere, so they organised a replacement fellow to do the flare-setting job. When we left Cairns we had a good south-easterly blowing. Now, with Cape Flattery being on the coast and normally blowing a gale, I had it in my head that we'd be landing into a south-easterly. It was only about a twenty-five-minute trip and when we arrived, there was a thin cloud cover at about 1000 feet. Of course, this happened back in the days when we didn't have GPS but the aircraft radar system was able to tell the difference between land and water. So I got myself over water by using that.

Then I let down—lost altitude—over the water, then came down under the cloud and over-flew the airstrip to check on things. Back then they had kerosene flares and I could see that the flares were all set out, ready for my landing. So I came around to position myself with the runway then on the final approach, at about 300 feet, suddenly all the flares went out. It was just like somebody had turned a light switch off. Every flare just disappeared like that—snap.

'God, what's going on here?' I said to Gary.

So straight away I went around. I put the props up and the power up and the undercarriage up and then, as soon as I did that, I got this horn going off … 'beep, beep, beep'. So there's this big red warning light flashing as we went back through the cloud. Of course, Gary the doctor, he's thinking about a previous trip when the fire alarms went off, so he's immediately on edge and saying, 'What's going on here? What's going on here?'

'I've got no idea,' I replied, which didn't inspire him with one iota of confidence, I can tell you.

Now, it wasn't that long before heading out on this trip that I'd been endorsed on this aeroplane. So while I knew the particular aircraft well, I wasn't completely familiar with it, if you understand my meaning. So I rechecked everything and realised that I still had full flaps down. Of course, as soon as I rectified that, the alarms stopped and everything settled down nicely … except Gary that is. For some strange reason he seemed to be shaking a fair bit.

So then we're back on top of this thin cloud layer again. 'Okay,' I said, 'I'll give it another go.'

As I said, it was night time. So it's back out over the water again, down under the cloud again, came back again, and over-flew the strip again to check the flares and, yes, all was right there. And it was while I was doing that I just happened to notice that about twenty miles away to the north-west of us there was a thunderstorm, and lightning started to flicker.

'Well, that's okay. That should be no problem,' I said. 'Let's attempt another landing.'

I came around again for the second attempt and as I was lining up to come in on final approach, I was getting blown around a bit. At the time I didn't realise it but what was happening was that the thunderstorm was pushing a local wind system in towards the aerodrome. So instead of me coming in against the south-easterly, as I'd assumed we would be doing, by now we were experiencing more of a north-westerly. Of course, I only found all this out later. So down we came again on final. I could see the flares, yes. I lined up, good. I could still see the flares, yes. In we came. Then at 300 feet, exactly the same thing happened again. Bang—all the flares went out. They disappeared.

I thought ... Oh, Jesus ...

Anyhow, we aborted the landing and up we went again. By this stage I sensed that Gary was feeling very uncomfortable about the whole situation.

But I thought, 'That's okay. Third time lucky.'

So I followed the same procedure for the third time and we came back in again. And suddenly the same thing happened. At 300 feet all the flares went out. Now I knew Cape Flattery quite well because I used to fly in and out of there pretty regularly and I knew there was a powerline we had to cross. So then I said to Gary, 'Well, I don't know. This time we're going in further. We've got to investigate this.'

Gary didn't answer me. He just sat there, stony faced and slightly grey. Anyhow, we continued on down and when the landing lights of the aeroplane lit up the powerlines and I still couldn't see any flares on the runway, I said, 'Well, that's it, out we go.'

'Great idea,' Gary said, suddenly sounding a little more enthusiastic. But then, just as we're going back through the cloud his enthusiasm turns to fear and he starts yelling out, 'The right-hand side motor's stopped. The right-hand side motor's stopped.'

'Well,' I said, 'if this aeroplane's climbing so well on one motor, I don't really care.'

Now actually Gary had gotten a bit overly nervous and jittery because what had happened was that we've got the strobe lighting on the end of the wings and, of course, when you go through cloud, visually it looks like the prop (propeller) has stopped. Basically, it's just an optical illusion, with the strobing effect and the cloud. That's all it was. But obviously Gary didn't realise that. He thought the motor had stopped.

'Don't worry about it,' I said. 'Let's just get out of here and go home.'

Then we were halfway back home to Cairns when Townsville calls up and says, 'Oh, the mine at Cape Flattery wants you to go back again.'

And I took one look at Gary and he nodded his head in a very determined manner and replied, 'Nope. Not again tonight. We'll go back at first light tomorrow morning.'

Anyway, we landed back at Cairns and the next morning we were up early and back out there and everything went like clockwork. We sorted out the problem at the mine and we also brought the lady back for her 'shopping trip'. And after that I think that some of Gary's waning faith in me as a pilot was restored … well, maybe just a little.

But, after thinking about it, I finally worked out what had gone wrong. See, the new fellow—the one who'd taken over the flare duties—when he saw the thunderstorm coming he became concerned that the north-westerly wind might blow the flares out. So to protect them from the wind, he placed the flares behind the witches hats—you know, those conical markers they use on airstrips and roads—and of course that meant when I came in to land and I hit a certain height and angle—which was the 300 feet level—the flares became hidden behind the witches hats. That's why they all suddenly disappeared on me.

So that solved the case of the disappearing flares.

Down the Lot

About twenty-five years ago my husband, Wayne, was a ranger out at Mootwingee Historic Site. That was before it became a National Park, later named Mutawintji. To give you some idea, Mootwingee is in north-western New South Wales, approximately halfway between Broken Hill and White Cliffs. And, as a ranger, my husband and another ranger looked after the district that went up to White Cliffs. So it was a big area.

But I was a city girl. I was a teacher and I'd come out to live there with our six-week-old baby. There was no television and no telephone and the only way of communication was by the two-way radio. So, as you might imagine, it was a very different life for a city girl, though I must add that it was certainly a very memorable time.

Basically, our only direct communications outside Mootwingee was with the School of the Air and the Royal Flying Doctor Service. The RFDS had medical sessions, mornings and late afternoons. That's when anyone could contact the Flying Doctor base in at Broken Hill and discuss any of their health issues with the doctor. It was exactly like a normal doctor's consultation but conducted over the two-way. So the doctor would listen to their symptoms then tell them what medicines they should self-administer from out of the medical chest that was provided for a small fee to each station property.

Of course, while these consultations were going on everybody else in the area was also tuned in, so everyone got to know all your intimate health problems. It was the same with the telegrams as well, see, because the telegrams were read out over the air every half hour—again, anybody could listen in. So then everyone got to know all your personal business as well as your intimate health problems. Then between the medical calls and the telegrams they used to have what was called the 'Galah Sessions'. That's when the lines were open so that anyone could have a chat to anyone else while, naturally, everybody else was listening in as well. So in such an isolated place, no one got away with anything and everyone out there knew everything about everybody else's business.

Initially, I was unaware of all this. Then when we first arrived at Mootwingee, the other ranger's wife came over and straight away she said to me, 'Oh,' she said, 'if you ever get thrush for God's sake don't call the Flying Doctor Service because everyone's always glued into their two-way radios and they'll have a great chuckle about it.'

Then she told me that, if I ever got thrush what number the medication was that I should use out of the medical chest we had.

'Oh fine,' I said, 'thanks for telling me.'

But, coming from the city, I still didn't quite believe her. I mean, you wouldn't, would you? That was until our six-week-old got his first cold and, even though it was nothing major, we radioed in to the RFDS doctor at Broken Hill for some medical advice. Then after that, whenever my husband went out on his rounds everyone would say, 'Oh, and how's the baby going? Is he over his cold yet?'

Anyhow, because there wasn't much in the way of other entertainment I must admit that even I started listening in to these sessions. And that brings me to the time I overheard a medical session on the two-way radio with a shearer on an outpost, and this shearer had some sort of a boil. Well, the doctor quizzed him about his diet and suggested that he, the shearer, and the rest of his shearing mates, should be eating more vegetables. Then the doctor said that the shearer should take a certain course of antibiotics from out of the medical chest. 'But only take as prescribed,' the doctor warned.

Now, I don't remember the exact name of the antibiotics that the doctor mentioned because, as I said, everything went by numbers. You know, the doctor would just say, 'Get bottle Number 65 and Number 28 out of your medical chest, take one tablet from each twice a day with meals, and that should fix the problem.'

Anyway, soon after the consultation between the shearer and the doctor had finished, the station manager's wife got on to the two-way radio and she called the shearer's cook, the one who was out at the outpost where the shearer with the boil was, and she started going crook on this cook. 'I hear that one of the shearers has got onto the doctor about his boil,' she said.

'Yes,' replied the cook.

Then the station manager's wife said, 'Look, I've told you lots and lots of times that you have to give the shearers vegetables. Feed them lots of vegetables. You can't just give them meat. You really have to cook them vegetables.'

And this is all happening over the two-way radio and, as I said, there I was, a city girl, and as much of an experience Mootwingee was, entertainment was a bit thin on the ground at times. But I'm just sitting back there listening to all this, with the station manager's wife going on and on, giving the shearer's cook a real ear full. And then in the end she said to the cook, 'Now, I want you to go to the medical chest and get those tablets that the doctor mentioned and you be responsible for giving them out to the shearer. And make sure you only give him the prescribed one tablet at a time because if you give him the whole bottle he'll more than likely down the lot in one go. You know these shearers—they'll try to get high on anything.'

And I just sat there laughing because I just had a vision of this shearer woofing into these antibiotics in an attempt to get high. Then I imagined that now the news was out, everyone in the whole area would be rifling through their medical chests also in search of these particular antibiotics.

Dr Clyde Fenton

In my last two books of flying doctor stories I wrongly named Clyde Fenton as Clive Fenton. Apparently this error has also been made by a number of historical museums and in other books of reference. I sincerely apologise for this error, and if you see Clyde's name presented wrongly in any other written form, please contact the publishers so that they can rectify the error.

Clyde Fenton was one of the first real 'Flying Doctors'. I say that because not only was he a doctor but he was also one of the very rare ones that actually flew the aeroplane. In fact, as a pilot during the war, he had an outstanding record and he was the Commanding Officer of No. 6 Communications Unit, out of Batchelor, which was about sixty kilometres south of Darwin.

Now, I don't know whether he had a plane when he first went to Katherine as a doctor or whether he bought the plane after he'd gone to Katherine. I somehow have a feeling it was after he'd gone to Katherine that he bought himself a little plane. This is all second-hand, of course, but they say that Clyde was a real daredevil in the air. When he was up in

Darwin he wasn't adverse to doing a few loop-d-loops over the airfield or taking a low skim over the outdoor picture theatre at night, to put the wind up the patrons, or even dive bombing groups who were out having a picnic.

Really, it sounded like he was a bit of a frustrated adventurer and so he was prepared to take some pretty huge risks with some of the flights that he did. Now, don't get me wrong: he was both a very good doctor and an excellent pilot and he saved many lives. I guess all those sorts of people took huge risks at some stage to get out into some of those more remote areas to help people who were in need. Still, it doesn't help anybody too much if they crash the plane on the way out or on the way back, does it? But that's the way it goes and sometimes you can't do too much about it.

Still, I find it interesting that when you look at plane crashes these days, very few people walk away from them, yet back then people did seem to survive more often, didn't they? Perhaps it had something to do with the lesser speeds they travelled at, because the planes back in those early days were made from not much more than wood and canvas so they'd rip apart upon contact with the ground, which was something that Clyde managed to do on a few occasions. I grew up at Humbert River Station, in the central-west of the Northern Territory, and I heard about the time when Clyde crashed a plane out on our neighbouring property of Victoria River Downs Station and the wreckage had to be packed up and put on the back of a truck and driven all the way back to Katherine.

It's also well documented that Clyde had a running battle with anything to do with 'the establishment'. In actual fact, he riled against anything to do with authority so, of course, just the mention of the Department of Civil Aviation, or DCA, had him seeing red. At one stage the DCA changed the licensing regulations and naturally Clyde steadfastly refused to go for this new licence. He considered it was just a whole lot of 'red tape, mumbo-jumbo and hog-wash'. Then when they threatened to take away his licence he flew over the house of the boss of the DCA and dropped a few flour bombs on the place. They even tried grounding him on a few occasions. But Clyde never ever took any notice. He simply continued on flying with his old licence. He'd just fly off anyway. I mean, nobody would dob him in if he was going out into the bush to help someone, would they?

So yes, Clyde was a real larrikin, alright. There's even been a couple of books written about him and his exploits. Just an example of one of those was the story about when he received the medal. That was when he was in Katherine; he was decorated with some sort of bravery award or other that came in the form of a medal. Anyway, because it had to do with 'authority' he didn't want anything to do with it. That's how anti-government and anti-establishment he was. But anyway, all these bigwigs still insisted on coming down to Katherine to present him with this special medal. So when they arrived at the Katherine Hospital, Clyde had all the staff lined up to greet them, and that included all the Aboriginal staff. And, much to the bigwigs' surprise and shock, Clyde had made mock tin replicas of the medal he was about to receive and he'd given one to every single member of the staff to wear on their uniform for the big occasion.

Of course, that didn't go over very well. But that was Clyde, and he was tremendously admired up in the Northern Territory, not only for the good he did as a doctor and pilot but also because of his larrikin ways. He was one of those that always tried to buck the system, and we tend to admire people like that in Australia, don't we?

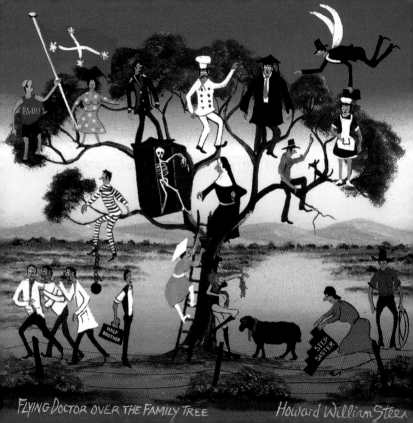

FLYING DOCTOR OVER THE FAMILY TREE

Howard William Steer

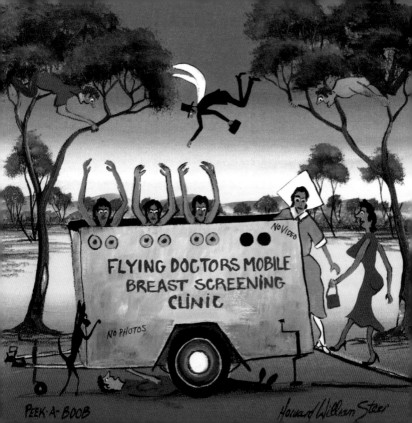

PEEK·A·BOOB   Howard William Steer

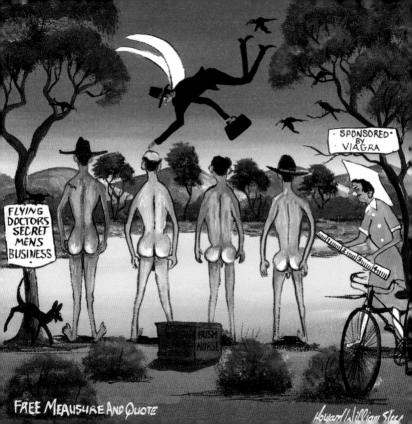

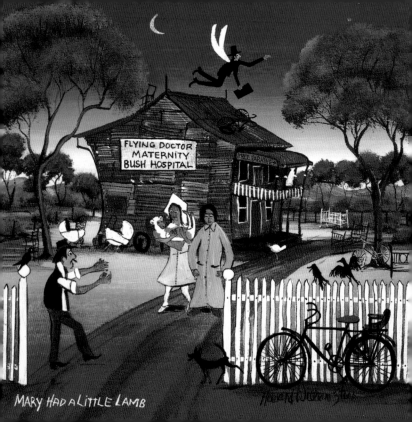

FLYING DOCTOR
MATERNITY
BUSH HOSPITAL

MARY HAD A LITTLE LAMB

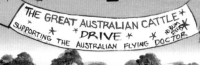

THE GREAT AUSTRALIAN CATTLE
DRIVE
SUPPORTING THE AUSTRALIAN FLYING DOCTOR

20 YEARS STOCKMANS HALL OF FAME

NO BUM STEER

DRIVING MISS DAISY

THE GREAT AUSTRALIAN CATTLE DRIVE
Howard William Steer

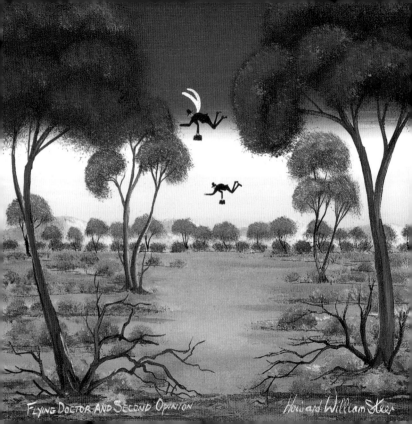

Flying Doctor And Second Opinion

Howard William Steer

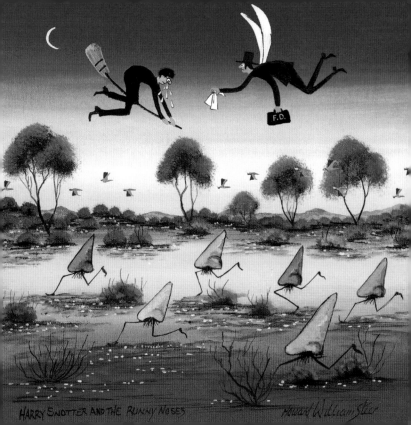

HARRY SNOTTER AND THE RUNNY NOSES   Howard William Steer

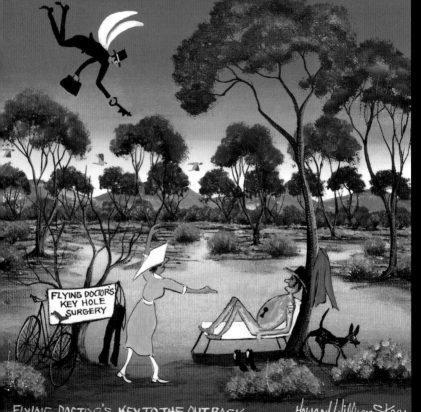

FLYING DOCTOR'S KEY TO THE OUTBACK

FLYING DOCTORS
KEY HOLE
SURGERY

Howard William Steer

From all Walks of Life

Back in 2000, around the time of the Sydney Olympics, we got a call one night to go on a retrieval up to Oodnadatta, in the far north-east of South Australia. But the thing was, we were getting mixed messages from our local contacts up there about what had actually happened. All they knew was that there'd been an accident somewhere out in the sticks but as yet they didn't have an exact location and they didn't know the extent of the injuries. Now, to my line of thinking, there was no good in us rushing off until we had confirmation as to what the real situation was. But our doctor had the retrieval equipment ready, the nurse ready, and so he wanted to get going as soon as possible.

We all have our areas of expertise in the Royal Flying Doctor Service, and with me being a pilot, basically the care of the aeroplane is my concern, and that includes fuelling. I knew that we could get fuel when we got to Oodnadatta but that meant pumping it out of drums, in the middle of the night, and I wanted to avoid that if possible, especially if it turned out to be an emergency. So I thought, well, I might go via Coober Pedy and take fuel on there, then I can go up to Oodnadatta and come straight back to Adelaide with any of the injured.

But the doctor said, 'No, I want to go straight to Oodnadatta.'

So that's what we did. Off we went to Oodnadatta. We'd found out by then that it was a two-vehicle accident and, being out in that desert area, we assumed it'd probably involve two four-wheel drive vehicles. Then, when we start the descent into Oodnadatta, I heard the doctor over the intercom saying that as soon as we landed he wanted to get hold of a vehicle and drive straight out to the accident site.

Oh, I thought, this spells disaster. Because, what really worried me was that it was a pitch black night and, to make matters worse, they still didn't know the exact whereabouts of the accident.

So I said to the nurse, 'Look, just don't go with them, otherwise we're going to end up with a retrieval team that's lost. Then we're going to have to get a search party to go looking for them and still there's the accident to attend to.'

Anyway, I landed at Oodnadatta and there was no further news. But the doctor remained adamant that he was going to organise transport out to wherever this accident had occurred. By then I'd decided that the safest thing for me to do was to camp out in the aircraft and wait and see what transpired. So they went into Oodnadatta—the nurse as well—and the last I heard was that they were going to try to organise lights—flares—to be moved to an airstrip on a station property, which they believed might be closer to the accident site. Now we didn't normally use the strip on that property at night, so once again I was pretty wary about going there.

Then at about daybreak a chap from the airport came out and when I asked what had happened he said 'Oh, they didn't go out. They're still here in Oodnadatta and they're having breakfast in at the hospital.'

When I got into the hospital I was told that the local people were also concerned about losing the RFDS retrieval team out in the desert and they'd strongly advised the doctor to stay at the hospital while some of the locals went in search of the accident. As luck would have it, they'd come across the two vehicles, away out in the sticks, and they were going to bring the people involved back to Oodnadatta. We were informed that there was one seriously injured person amongst them.

Then while we were having breakfast they told me the exact location where the accident had occurred and I said, 'Look, to save them coming all the way back to Oodnadatta, how about we radio them and say that we'll meet them at Dalhousie Springs.'

And that's what we did and, believe it or not, just as I landed the plane at Dalhousie Springs, they arrived. But while they were loading the patient I spoke to the guy who drove the vehicle out in search of the accident. He was a part-Aborigine who'd grown up in the area and he'd spent some time in the Army. So he was an experienced bushman who knew the area very well, and I said to him, 'How did you go driving out to the accident site then back to Dalhousie?'

'Well,' he said, 'actually I got lost a couple of times but I didn't tell the others, just in case they'd panic.'

So the whole retrieval may well have been a real shemozzle. But thankfully the doctor had taken the expert advice of the locals and stayed put in Oodnadatta. Anyway, we transferred the injured patient to Adelaide. But he was okay. His condition wasn't as bad as was first believed.

But this is the thing; see, you've got various people from all walks of life involved in all our operations. Not only the doctors, nurses and pilots, but there's also all the people on the ground. And it's important that everyone sticks to their area of expertise and be very clear about where they stand. Very clear. The last thing you need is for a pilot to be telling a nurse how to treat a patient or for a doctor to be telling a local how to get to an accident site. It just doesn't work. So essentially I think the organisational side of things within the RFDS is very good. The way it's set up; there's no grey areas.

Anyway, that was quite an unusual one for us really, because that type of accident is normally handled out of Port Augusta. But we're always there to back each other up, just in case of aeroplane or personnel unavailability. And just as well, because with a lot more inexperienced people travelling out into the outback, they're extremely lucky to have an organisation like the RFDS so readily and expertly available.

Gymkhanas

My name's John Lynch. I'm the CEO of the Royal Flying Doctor Service's Central Operations and, if you've got a minute, I've got a few stories to tell. Now, due to the isolation of the outback, the local gymkhanas are a huge social occasion for station people and the like who otherwise would rarely have the chance to get together. And of course, while everyone's in the one place, we usually set up a tent to run a medical clinic so that people can have a health check or whatever. Now I'm particularly talking about the blokes here because, you know, while they're all in town for the gymkhana, it's an opportune time to grab them where there's less focus on them having to make a special appointment and come all the way into town to visit the doctor. You know what blokes are like.

So it'll quite often be, 'Well, mate, if you go across to see the doctor for a health check, I may as well go too.'

'Okay then, let's all go.' That sort of thing.

And also the gymkhanas are usually designed as a fundraiser for the Royal Flying Doctor Service. So I've got a few stories about gymkhanas, and I guess that the first of these stories goes to demonstrate the huge excitement that a gymkhana generates. Now, we had a new doctor who'd never been to a gymkhana and, as I said before, a gymkhana is one of those rare opportunities when everyone gets together. What's more, you must appreciate that some of these young, single fellers and girls might never have had a lot of regular social contact, particularly with the opposite sex. So when they get together they sometimes get pretty—how can I say it—'frisky'.

Anyway, one of our new doctors went up to this town to run the on-course medical clinic. He arrived on the morning of the gymkhana and the first thing he did was that he went over to the nursing station to introduce himself. 'Hello,' he said, 'I'm doctor so-and-so from the Flying Doctor Service.'

'Yep, no worries,' said the nurse. They all knew his name.

'Oh, I almost forgot,' said the doctor, and he handed over a package to the nurse. 'There you go; I brought along some condoms, just in case they're needed.'

And the nurse looked at him and she said, 'I reckon you might be a bit too late, doctor. The mob got into town last night and they've been having a hell of a good time ever since.'

So the party had already begun.

Then, after he handed over the condoms, this new doctor went off and he set up a little tent to do his medical checks and some of these younger kids, of course they run around all day and they have busters and so forth and so they're always going to the doctor to get their grazes fixed up. Anyhow, one young kid arrives with a grazed knee and the doctor's taking a look at it when a call comes over the loudspeaker: 'Could the Flying Doctor come urgently to the finishing post.'

Instantly of course he thinks, 'Dear me, someone's fallen off a horse and injured themselves badly.'

So the doctor tried to hurry up with this kid but he's interrupted by another call over the loudspeaker: 'The Flying Doctor is very urgently required at the finishing post.'

'Look,' the doctor said to the kid, 'there's an emergency so I'll just stick a band-aid over your graze and if it's still bothering you, come back later and I'll sort it out properly.'

Then he quickly stuck a band-aid on the kid, grabbed his medical bag and he took off like a rocket, out of the tent, through the crowd, under the fence, out onto the track and over to the finishing post, all the while preparing himself for the worst. Then, when he got to the finishing post, he ran up to the bloke with the microphone and he said, 'Yes ... (puff) ... yes ... I'm ... (puff) ... the Flying Doctor. Where's the emergency?'

And the bloke on the microphone said, 'Where the hell have you been? We've been waiting for you to come and draw the bloody raffle.'

So I guess that goes to show the social intricacies of a gymkhana, and what the responsibilities and the expectations sometimes are of the people from the Flying Doctor Service. And we're ever so lucky that those outback people are also just fundamentally open and honest with you. In many ways it's as if we're one big family. It's like that old bloke in one of the original promotional videos, or was it a film. But anyway, I saw this footage of an old weather-beaten bush character. He's right out in the outback and, you know, he's got the typical old battered hat—pushed back with sweat stains all around the brim—that'd been worn for that many years it'd become part of the personality. And even though you don't see it much today because of the health risks, he's got the roll-your-own cigarette, hanging out the side of his mouth, he's wearing the standard chequered shirt, with a tin of tobacco stuck in the top pocket, sleeves rolled up, the R M Williams riding boots and the well-worn jeans, and they asked him, 'What does the Flying Doctor mean to you?'

And the old feller, he said, 'The Flying Doctor?' Then he pushed back his hat and scratched his forehead, while he had a bit of a think. Then, with just the slightest glint in his eye, he answered, 'Well,' he said, 'without the Royal Flying Doctor Service I'd reckon there'd be a hell of a lotta dead people livin' out here.'

And, again, that's just so typical of those people. Wonderful people. Wonderful humour.

But while we're talking about gymkhanas and wonderful fellers with wonderful humour, I must mention Johnny Watkins, 'Watto' as he's known. Watto just happens to have found the recipe for that weather-beaten outback look. He's a terrific fellow and just one of the greatest supporters of the RFDS. In fact, he's a wonderful supporter of the bush. Watto was the Elders man and auctioneer throughout the north of South Australia so naturally he landed the job as the auctioneer at the William Creek Gymkhana (Races), which is another great fundraising event for the RFDS. It was my first time up at William Creek and a lot of people from Port

Augusta got together and formed a syndicate to buy horses for the day in an attempt to try and win some cup or ribbon or other. Of course, much of the money from the buying of horses goes to the Flying Doctor Service.

Anyway, being the CEO of the RFDS in that area, I thought that maybe I should buy a horse as well. Well, the truth be known, Watto very strongly suggested that I should buy a horse. Now I didn't have a clue about horses but Watto stepped in and he told me, in the strictest of confidences, that the next horse to be auctioned was a 'real beauty'. Apparently it had some sort of 'impeccable breeding'. Even the name Bart Cummings may have been mentioned. I forget now but Watto described it as being the 'sleeper' of the entire gymkhana.

'Okay,' I said, 'I'll bid for it.'

'Don't worry,' said Watto, 'I'll make sure you get it at a reasonable price.'

So the bidding begins and Watto calls out, 'Who can start me off with twenty dollars?'

Well, I stick my hand up to put in my bid, fully expecting to get the horse for twenty dollars; it sounded like a bargain to me, even being a mug punter. But then Watto said, 'I've got thirty dollars. Who can better thirty for this beautifully bred horse? Yes, forty dollars ... fifty dollars ... Yes, sixty dollars to Johnny Lynch the CEO. Seventy dollars ... eighty dollars ... one hundred and twenty dollars to Johnny Lynch.' And I'm just standing there. I haven't even moved a muscle. I only bid twenty dollars on this nag and the next thing Watto's telling me that I've just bid $120 for it.

Anyway, I finally end up getting this 'beautifully bred horse'—this dead cert—for something like $150 and the only thing I'm dead certain about is that I was the only one to have put in a single bid. No one else even bothered. But anyway, I've got this horse, so I said to Watto, 'What do I do now?'

And he said, 'You need to go over and pay for it.'

So I started to walk across to where I had to pay for the horse and this young Aboriginal fellow come up and he said, 'You got a jockey, Boss?'

I said, 'A jockey? No.' I hadn't even thought about a jockey.

'Well,' he said, 'who's ridin' the horse?'

I said, 'I don't know.'

'I'm a jockey,' he said. 'I'm the best.'

'Oh, are you?' I said.

He said, 'You want me to be your jockey?'

I said, 'Well, okay, then.' I said, 'If you want to be my jockey, then you've got the job.'

'Yeah, Boss,' he said, 'I'm the best. You won't regret it.' Then he said, 'Well, we'd better put the horse in the race.'

'Yeah, no worries,' I said. 'What race will we go in?'

He said, 'All of 'em.'

And so the relationship had been struck, and this young Aboriginal fellow made it clear that because I was the owner of the horse, I was to be known as the 'Boss', and he was to be called the 'Boy', as, apparently that's what jockeys are called by the owners. And he rode that horse—that dead cert—in every event that was on. There was the peg race. Then they had the distance race. Then there was a 400-metre race. Then there was some bloody race where the horse went around and around in ever decreasing circles. And we never got a prize; never even got a ribbon. Not even a placing. Nothing. In fact, there was one race where the jockey—the 'Boy'—had to go and pick up pegs then put them into a barrel, and I said to him after the race, 'If they have that race again,' I said, 'is there any chance that the horse can ride you because the horse is too bloody slow and you keep missing the barrel.'

But, you know, he was a terrific little fellow, this young Aborigine. I think he said he was nineteen, and he rode in every race. And he never missed me because after each disastrous event he always came across to explain to me what had gone wrong with the horse. Then I'd thank him for the explanation and I'd pay him a couple of bob for the ride.

'Thanks, Boss,' he'd say. 'We'll have better luck next time.'

But we never did.

Hats off

Well, I've certainly had a lot more experiences since your first book of *Great Australian Flying Doctor Stories* came out, way back in 1999. So yes, I can give you a few more stories and, mind you, these are from a doctor's point of view, of course. One that knocked me for six was an amazing story of survival stemming from an accident that happened in the Carnarvon National Park, which is in south-eastern Queensland, sort of, north-east of Charleville. It's near a place called Injune.

Okay, it was a week day, about mid-day, when I got a call on the HF radio from a ranger fellow out in the Carnarvon National Park. He said that he'd been driving around the park and he'd come across an accident. A utility vehicle was down in a roadside drain with the male driver slumped over the steering wheel. The driver was unconscious. Because there were no other vehicles about, the fellow that reported the accident assumed it'd been a single vehicle accident. So I advised him what to do until we got up there. I also requested that I be met at the nearest airstrip, at an ETA (estimated time of arrival) to be advised, and for them to be prepared to take us, in one of their vehicles, out to the accident site. The driver chap was still in the car at this time and he still remained slumped over the steering wheel.

So we flew up to the Carnarvon National Park and landed at the Mount Moffatt airstrip, where the park's people met us in a vehicle. They then took us from there, with all our equipment, up to where they'd found the vehicle. Upon arrival at the scene of the accident my suspicions were immediately aroused because, firstly, there were no skid marks and, secondly, there was no sign of there being any damage to the vehicle. When we got the fellow out of his vehicle, my primary assessment suggested that he was in some sort of shock. At that stage I didn't know which sort of shock it was. Anyway, I got a large bore intravenous cannula into him and gave him a couple of litres of fluid fairly quickly, and this improved his situation somewhat. I then did a secondary survey, which is a head-to-toe survey, of his wellbeing. Things did not look good: his face had been badly pushed in; his chest was a bit suspect. I estimated that his belly was full of blood, and he had bilateral mid-shaft of femurs, with both sticking out at right angles. That's his thigh bone. He also had a fractured forearm.

By that stage I'd resuscitated him and he was able to talk to us, just a little, and he managed to inform us as to what had happened. As it turned out, there was just him and his dog and he'd been cutting down a tree for firewood in the National Park, which was illegal—though that was the least of our concerns at that stage. While he was cutting a tree, it had fallen on him, trapping him underneath it. So that's when he had sustained all these injuries I've just described. Then, somehow—and I don't know how—he'd worked his way out from underneath the tree. His ute was parked across the flat and he must've crawled his way over to the ute, a distance of a couple of hundred yards. He then put the dog in the back of his utility vehicle and made sure the dog was safe, then he somehow managed to get himself in the front of the vehicle. How he managed to do this, in his condition, I would not have a clue.

He then drove the vehicle—it was a manual—to a nearby homestead, where he knew there was a telephone. When he arrived at the homestead he couldn't raise anyone. Nobody was at home. So he went back out onto the road where he had obviously at some stage just passed out from the loss of blood. That's when he put his vehicle in the roadside ditch, which was where the ranger fellow had come across him, slumped over the steering wheel.

So we stabilised him as best we could. Then we put him onto the back of a vehicle and they took him over a very, very rough road, back to the aeroplane. And, you wouldn't believe this, but the whole way back to the aeroplane he cracked jokes like nobody's business and I'm sure it wasn't just from the happy juice I'd administered to him.

Anyway, we put him in the aeroplane and we took him down to Royal Brisbane Hospital. He had a laparotomy that night—that's opening up his belly—and basically they found that he had a ruptured liver as well as all the other injuries I've previously described.

I'm afraid I didn't follow up on the dog because I had my hands full, assessing and stabilising the patient. But as far as I was concerned I'd have to say 'Hats off' to this fellow. Because let's focus on the injuries that he would've sustained when the tree fell on him. As a summary: his face had been quite severely damaged. He had a fractured forearm. He had bilateral mid-shaft of femurs; in other words both sides of his femurs were broken at right angles, which meant that they were sticking out at right angles. He had a belly full of blood, which later on proved to be from a ruptured liver. His chest was suspect at the time, possibly from the blood in the belly pushing up to the diaphragm. I wasn't sure how, at that early stage, but he was still able to maintain his respiratory drive okay, so I didn't have to ventilate him.

Now considering his condition I ask you, with all those injuries, first of all, how did he get out from under the tree? Then how did he manage to crawl the couple of hundred yards across the ground to his ute? Following that, how did he manage to get into the ute and then drive the vehicle to the homestead, keeping in mind that it was a manual drive.

In my time as a doctor, it's one of the greatest survival stories that I have known. And the people at the Royal Brisbane Hospital, they put him back together and he could walk again after all that. In fact, I last saw him walking down the street in Injune.

Heroes of the Outback

What you've got to take into consideration is that it's not just the vast distances we in the Royal Flying Doctor Service have to cover, but also the many, many miles that some of our constituents have to travel to get anywhere. Now this notion of distance may seem inconceivable for someone who is living in a city, where all the amenities are so close. But that's not the way it is out there, in the more isolated areas. For example, take the time we had to cancel a medical clinic—at short notice—from out of our operations at Port Augusta. This was a few years ago now so I can't quite remember where the clinic was originally going to be held and nor can I remember what the exact reason was as to why we had to cancel it. It could've been due to bad weather, which is the most likely reason, or it may have even been aircraft or crew unavailability. Those things happen sometimes. But anyway, the issue was that we were forced to cancel the clinic, and as soon as that decision had been made we let everyone know.

Then shortly after we notified everyone of the cancellation I got a call from a woman who used to attend this particular clinic, whenever the need arose. 'I've just arrived at our front gate and my husband's called to say that you've cancelled the medical clinic,' she said.

'Yes,' I said, 'that's right.'

'Why did you do that?'

'Well,' I said, 'I'm not exactly sure but I can find out and radio you back, if you like.'

'Oh,' she said, 'there's no need for that but I would've liked to have known a little bit earlier.'

Now, if you lived in the city your normal reaction would be to say, 'Well, that shouldn't be too much of a problem; just turn around and go back inside your house.' Because if you do live in the city and you've walked out the door and you've just arrived at your front gate and your husband's called out to tell you that the doctor's now unavailable, then you'd just turn around and go back inside, wouldn't you? It's that easy.

Anyhow, this woman, she said to me, 'Yeah well, I guess that I'll just have to turn around and go back home now, but it seems to be an enormous waste of time.'

'Well,' I said, 'I sincerely apologise but it's still only nine o'clock in the morning.'

'Yes,' she said, 'it may still only be nine o'clock in the morning but I've already travelled well over sixty kilometres, along a dirt track, and that's just from my back door to the front gate of our property.'

And that put it into some sort of perspective. You know, because of the distances that some of these people have to travel—just to reach their own front gate—a cancellation like that is not a simple thing.

So you have to admire people like that, particularly the women. Take our Consumer Network Group. It's a wonderful way of engaging with the actual people we serve. It's made up of predominantly females and we get together every now and then for face-to-face meetings to discuss how the RFDS can better serve its constituents. We're actually reinvigorating it now, which is very exciting, because you get everyone talking about things like the services they're receiving, and the frequency they get them, and the freedom of access and, you know, things like: are we meeting their requirements? Can we do it better? Is there something else we should be looking at?

Now, I'm not saying that we can always rectify all these matters because, as you may be able to imagine, there are huge logistical problems in servicing such vast areas of this continent. Like I said about that woman before—it's not like she could simply just turn around and go back home and get on with her day as if nothing had happened.

And so, when I get to talk to the many people that go to these Consumer Network Group meetings, I'm always reminded of that John Williamson song, 'Woman on the Land'. I don't know whether you've ever heard it or not. It goes something like, 'So I propose a toast to the mothers that we know. Proud to be the better half who really run the show ... To our hero—the woman on the land.' It's a magnificent song. Anyhow, I learned the words for one particular Consumer Network Group meeting because, you know, the last thing we want is for our constituents to reach a point where they're just a recorded number. They're more than that. They're people. They're human beings. And those women, and in actual fact everyone we serve, they are the real heroes of the outback.

Of course, it's not just the Royal Flying Doctor Service who supports them. There are many other organisations involved. And also, of course, the people themselves are also extremely supportive of each other, perhaps sometimes a little too over zealously. There's one occasion that always tickles me: I remember when I was with one of the doctors during a phone-in medical session. They used to happen over the air, twice daily. The first session was at eight o'clock in the morning, before the School of the Air program started, and the second was at four o'clock in the afternoon, after School of the Air had finished. They were timed that way because the mums were often fairly busy, not just supervising their children during their classes but also helping run the property, as well as attending to the normal 'womanly' chores of washing, cooking, cleaning, plus the multitude of other tasks they take on. Like I said, real heroes of the outback.

Now, what you've got to appreciate is that these medical sessions were open sessions. Anyone could listen in, and they quite often did. It was an easy way for everyone to find out how everyone else was going. So this time the doctor opened the radio and initially he registered who was out there. Then once everyone was registered, he went back to the first person. He gave her call sign and the lady replied with, 'I'm just a bit concerned about little Johnny.'

'Oh yes,' replied the doctor, 'can you tell me his symptoms?'

'Well, Doctor, he's got such and such.' And she described little Johnny's symptoms.

Then before the doctor could even answer, one of the lady's neighbours cut in, over the radio, and said, 'Oh, I can tell you exactly what's wrong with him.'

And I thought that that showed the real essence of the bush: you know, how even if these people are hundreds of miles apart, they're not only comfortable talking about their own personal issues to a doctor, while everyone else was listening in, but they were also willing to put in their sixpence worth if they thought they could help each other out.

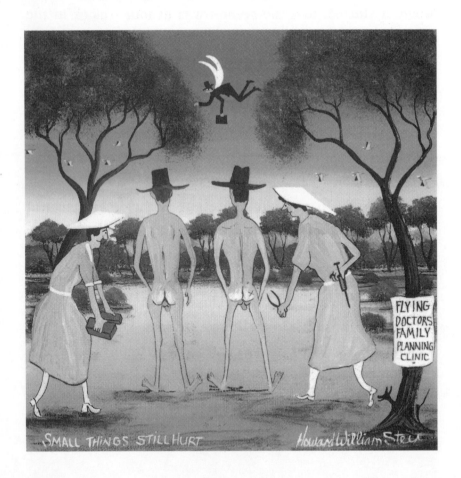

SMALL THINGS STILL HURT   Howard William Steer

I Was the Pilot

I've just been reading your second book of flying doctor stories—*More Great Australian Flying Doctor Stories*—and in that book there's one particular story called 'Blown Away'. Now you're not going to believe this but I was the pilot that was mentioned in that story and in actual fact, over my time in the Royal Flying Doctor Service, it's one of my all-time favourite stories as well. So, would you like to hear the story from the pilot's side of the event?

If you don't mind, I've sort of written bits and pieces of it down and I'd like to read it to you more or less as I've written it. So, okay, here goes.

One of my favourite stories happened not long after I started with the Flying Doctor Service. So that must've been about 1990 or thereabouts. Anyway, I was working at Port Hedland at the time and we received a call from a family who were driving along the Canning Stock Route.

Now, I'm presuming here that everyone knows where the Canning Stock Route is. If not, I'd just like to relate a brief overview because it will give the readers a clearer picture of the desolation of the situation. The Canning is an old stock route that runs a distance of 1820 kilometres along a series of wells through the central deserts of Western Australia, from

Halls Creek, in the north, right down to near Wiluna, which is just west of Meekatharra. I'm not sure what it's like today, but originally there were supposed to be something like fifty-one wells, or watering points, along the length of the stock route. Then over the stock route's historic period, from when the track was being surveyed and then during the following years when droving was taking place, the records tell us that there were something like ten murders, a number of inflicted woundings and several deaths from internal complications of—and I quote—'unknown origin'. These murders, woundings and deaths from unknown origins involved both white and indigenous people.

Also there were and still are countless sand ridges. And I'll quote again here—'According to Dr J. S. Bard, over one particular section of 470 miles, some 730 sand ridges lay along the stock route, containing enough material to cover the country evenly with sand to a depth of three feet. The biggest sand ridges are between Wells 41 and 42. When formed they are approximately a mile apart, averaging sixty feet in height, with a base of about 320 feet.'

So, if you can calculate that back to the figures we use these days, that might just give you some idea as to what the country out there is like. And while droving no longer takes place along the Canning these days, it's a favourite journey-cum-adventure for many four-wheel drivers.

Anyhow, these people were camped near Well 33, which was right out, oh, it's probably only about 200 kilometres from the Northern Territory border. So it's fairly well east.

And they were travelling in convoy with another couple, who were also in a four-wheel drive vehicle. Anyhow, their young daughter, who was about nine or ten years old, climbed about the only tree that was out in that part of the desert and the branch broke and she fell down and broke what I believe was her arm. In your story, the storyteller thought that she'd fractured one of her thighs. So I stand corrected on that point. Mind you, it was a long time ago.

Now, as luck would have it, they were reasonably close to an old airstrip. The only trouble was that the strip hadn't been used for a very long time. Now, I'm trying to remember just what the name of that particular strip was. No, sorry, I can't remember just off hand. Anyway, it was overgrown with short, low bushes, maybe up to something like a metre high. So, as I said, it hadn't been used for a fair while.

We got the call the night before we went out there and, of course, naturally there were no landing lights on the strip out there or anything so we had to wait until first light to head off. At that point of time, with the airstrip being so overgrown, it was impossible for us to land anyway. But all through the night these people and their other companions worked by their car headlights, clearing the bushes with shovels and spades and whatnot.

Then I flew out of our Port Hedland Base just before first light in an attempt to arrive at the remote airstrip just on first light. When I arrived, the strip still looked pretty rough but it looked landable so I was willing to give it a try. These people, they'd set up a fire with the smoke to show me the wind direction. Anyhow, I landed the plane on this makeshift strip and we successfully picked up the little girl and her mother and took them back to Port Hedland, where the little girl received further necessary treatment. So that was a very satisfying retrieval.

I think that the people were from Victoria somewhere, and later on we got a lovely letter back from the little girl thanking us for what we did. Then along with her letter the girl's parents sent some lovely photos of, you know, the girl lying in the back of the car and the airstrip before they cleared it and then after they'd cleared it and also of the aeroplane coming in to land. But it must've been a hell of a job to clear the airstrip, which had to be about 1000 metres long. I mean, that's quite a lot of work they did, and, as I said, they worked all night.

But in her letter the little girl also told us how her broken limb had healed and how that everything was now fine, thanks to us. And that really warms your heart. So, there's just another side of that story—'Blown Away'—that you related in your book *More Great Australian Flying Doctor* stories, and really, as I said, it is one of my very favourites.

If only

I can honestly say that the three years I spent in Alice Springs, while I was flying for the Flying Doctor Service, was the most enjoyable and rewarding experience in my life. I had an absolute ball. Though, in saying that, of course everything didn't always go as well as I would have wanted it to go. And unfortunately this was the one particular case that still gets to me because, you know, if only the weather conditions had been different, this patient is one that we could've very possibly saved.

Anyhow, it was three o'clock in the afternoon when I got the call to fly out to Tennant Creek and pick up this little kid. She was a young eleven-year-old girl. The only trouble was that there were storms about everywhere. And, mind you, in Alice Springs you do get some very big storms, especially when it's the wet season up north. Anyway, these storms were a bit too big for my liking. Still and all, the situation sounded very serious so I told them that I'd have another think about it before I made a final call. As you may well know, anything to do with the flying part of the RFDS is up to the pilot, and the pilot not only has to think of the safety aspects of every trip he makes, he's also got to keep in mind that he's responsible for a couple of million dollars worth of aeroplane plus the lives of the doctor and nurse who may be accompanying him on such a trip.

So I did have a good think about it, balancing the safety aspects of such a flight against the desperate need of the child and, based on the fact that it would be in the dead of night when we returned and we had no weather radar, I made my final decision. So I got back in touch with Tennant Creek and said, 'No, I won't go. It's too risky. But I'll definitely be in the air as soon as the storms dissipate.'

Then, the first chance we got, we went. I think we left about one o'clock in the morning—this is up in Tennant Creek—to pick up this young girl.

When we got to Tennant Creek the doctor took one look at the poor little kid and he pulled me aside and said, 'Gee, she's as good as gone. What's more, we can't do anything more for her in Alice Springs than what I can do for her here, in Tennant Creek.' He said, 'There's only two options: one is to take her straight down to Adelaide and the other is to get her to Darwin as soon as humanly possible.'

Darwin was closest, of course, but, as I said, it was the wet season, which was why the storms were so bad in Alice Springs. Anyhow, just in case, I rang up and got the weather report for Darwin and they told me that it was okay for the present.

'Right-o,' I said to the doctor. 'Darwin it is.'

So we went helter-skelter to Darwin and because of the restrictive weather conditions and the emergency of the case, I was the only light aircraft to be given permission to land in Darwin that day. Anyway, you wouldn't believe it but, the poor little child died just when we got there. We were still on the tarmac. A girl it was—a dear little eleven-year-old girl, just a kid.

And that case still gets to me because if only I'd been able to fly up to Tennant Creek the night before, who knows what might've happened. But the weather was against us. Everything was against us. And the thing is, as I said, as a pilot you're not only responsible for yourself and the aeroplane but there's also the nurses and the doctors that you've got to think about. And each and every one of us has to ensure that we're there to fight another day.

But in the three years I was in Alice Springs that was only one, you know, that I had any doubt on. Yes, of course, others have died, which was unfortunate, though there was more than a good chance that they would've died anyway. But that little girl was the only one I have any doubt about. And it still gets to me, even to this day.

In Double Quick Time

I've got a story here that has quite an amusing aspect to it. See, from time to time, the Flying Doctor Service used to get the occasional complaint about how long it took us to get out to some of these remote places to pick people up. You know, along the lines of, 'Gees, youse took yer bloody time', sort of thing.

But of course we couldn't be everywhere at the same time and, mind you, we did have vast distances to cover. And then of course we're all human beings so, naturally, when someone's seriously ill or injured or something, well, we all get a bit upset and stressed when help doesn't arrive immediately.

Anyway, this is when I was flying the King Air aeroplanes, so it'd be back in the early 1990s, and on this particular occasion we'd been up to one of the Aboriginal communities— it was either Kowanyama or Pormpuraaw—to pick up someone. So we were on the way back home with this patient. At that stage of the game our base in at Cairns received an emergency call from a certain property—Bolwarra—to say that they had a stockman who'd fallen off his horse and he had a very badly broken ankle. The people from the property had spoken to the doctor in at our Cairns base and the doctor had said, 'Well, we'd better do an "evac" and get the feller out of there as quick as possible.'

Now, unbeknown to the people on the property of Bolwarra, we turned out to be flying virtually right over the top of them when we got the message. So within fifteen minutes of their call I had the King Air landing at their airstrip. And they were amazed. 'For heaven's sake,' they said, 'you wouldn't get a faster service from the road ambulance in the city.'

So we reckoned we'd made up for any perceived 'tardiness' we might've had in the past, just on that one 'evac'. You know, to be able to produce the aeroplane, in front of an anxiously waiting group of people and a seriously injured stockman, within ten or fifteen minutes of them calling Cairns was just about unheard of. It was just pure luck, of course. As I said, we just happened to be returning from picking up another patient and were basically right over the top of the place.

But the poor bloke—the stockman—he was really in a bad way. He had an extremely bad compound fracture, where the bone was actually protruding through the skin of his ankle. It was a shocker. Very distressing, really. But it was just typical of these outback people. I tell you, they're as tough as nails and with an amazing sort of resilience, because when the stockman was asked, 'Is it hurting?' he gave a wince and replied, 'Oh, it itches a bit.'

Anyhow, we got him back to Cairns in pretty quick time and he didn't lose his ankle or his foot. Mind you, I'm not sure he was able to run as fast as he had in the past but they were able to fix his foot up. So he could walk and that was great.

In the ...

When I first went up to Cape York to work with the Australian Inland Mission, there was a story going around that went something like this. Now, you know how cooks have the reputation of being temperamental people. Well, one of the station properties had this rather large cook who, when he got into a 'paddy' about anything, would grab a book and go out and plonk himself down in the outhouse toilet and, depending on the gravity of the paddy he was in, maybe not come out for anything up to a couple of hours.

Of course, back then there weren't any septic systems in those remote areas so the type of toilets they used were the 'long-drop' type. For those of you that may not know, the long-drop toilet is basically, you know, a wooden box type of thing with a hole in the top where the seat goes, and that's all placed over a very deep hole, which is where all the 'waste' goes. For privacy, it's surrounded by a few sheets of corrugated iron, a roof and a wooden door. That particular style of toilet was well suited to Cape York because, being an old mining area, the actual toilet itself was simply plonked down over an old mine shaft, which saved a lot of digging.

Anyway, early one morning this cranky cook got his knickers in a knot about something or other, so he grabbed a book and went out and plonked himself down on the toilet. Unfortunately, the white ants must've been very busy of late because when he sat down the toilet crumbled from under him and he, in turn, disappeared down this old mine shaft. Actually, you could liken it to what happened to Alice in the book *Alice in Wonderland*, except that this cook really landed in the ... well, you can imagine what he landed in, can't you?

Now, seeing that all the ringers and stockmen and that who worked on this station property were well aware of the cook's temperamental nature, when he hadn't come out of the toilet by breakfast time they didn't worry too much, and they just went ahead and helped themselves. Even by morning tea there was still only some semi-mild concern. But by lunch time, some hours later, these stockmen were starting to get pretty hungry and even though the cook wasn't what you'd call 'a gourmet specialist', at least he dished up a pretty hearty meal.

Anyway, one of the younger ringers drew the short straw and he got landed with the job of going over to the outhouse to check on the situation. So he wandered over to the long-drop, knocked on the wooden door and said, 'Cookie, are yer okay?'

There was no answer so the ringer knocked a little louder, 'Hey, Cookie, we're getting hungry.'

Still no answer. Then, just as the ringer was about to walk away, he thought he heard a very faint voice. This's a bit odd, thought the ringer and he called out for his mates to come over and offer a second opinion. They all gathered around the outhouse. 'Hey, Cookie!' they shouted.

'Help,' came the distant reply.

So they broke down the toilet door and that's when they discovered that the cook had disappeared down the old mine shaft.

'Hey, Cookie, are yer down there?'

'Yes,' came the echo.

Anyway, while someone went over to the homestead to get on the radio and call the Flying Doctor, the stockmen knocked down the outer, corrugated iron, toilet structure and then they got the ropes and all the rest of it and they hooked up a 'windlass'—a winch lift—to haul the cook out.

Even though the cook had been extricated from his predicament by the time the Flying Doctor arrived, the poor chap was still in rather a smelly state. But the doctor, being the professional that he was, checked the cook out to make sure that he was okay and luckily, apart from a very bruised ego, the cook had survived the experience without too many injuries at all. But just to be on the safe side, the doctor decided to give him a course of antibiotics, because of the, you know, the particular situation he'd been in. And as the story went, the cook lost a little of his temperamental sharpness after that event and even when he did throw a paddy, just before he'd storm out of the kitchen he'd announce to all and sundry, 'Won't be long, fellers.'

In the Beginning

I got into flying in quite an odd sort of way, really. Back during World War II, my older brother, Bill, had been a flying officer in the Royal Australian Air Force (RAAF), No. 13 Squadron, up in Darwin. He was flying Hudsons. Then on 19 February 1942 he got shot down over the Timor Sea and was listed as missing. And that event changed the course of my life really, because at that stage I'd put my age up and had already enlisted in the Army. But then, after Bill went missing, I resolved to get into the Air Force when I'd reached their required age of eighteen.

Finally, after being accepted into the RAAF, my initial training was held at Victor Harbor, which is south of Adelaide, in South Australia. After that I was posted to Narrandera, in south-western New South Wales, where I was instructed in elementary flying in the Tiger Moths. After eight months there, I returned to South Australia, this time to Mallala, where I built up 140 flying hours. I was then deemed ready for service with the RAAF.

After the war had ended, I went back on the land and although I maintained my private licence through the Aero Club of South Australia, my flying career basically went on hold. But even then I still continued to explore any possible opportunities towards a flying career. To that end, in 1959 I purchased my own Cessna and started up as a charter pilot, based in the far west of New South Wales, at a place called Wilcannia. My main work out there came through stock firms like Elders, Goldsbrough Mort and Dalgety's. But then the drought of 1963 put paid to all that and so I adapted my aircraft and began selling pest control products throughout South Australia, Queensland and the Northern Territory. As it turned out, there was an untapped market in those outback areas and flying the Cessna was a great way to reach them, because in those days you could land just about anywhere. So even though I wasn't a salesperson by nature, because of the accessibility I had, I still had great success.

Then in 1965 I sold my aircraft to Ross Aviation and joined their firm in Adelaide. Ross Aviation was a sales and charter company so I had a combination of work, with demonstrating and selling aircraft plus flying charter. That job took me all over Australia, and from Adelaide I was offered a job in Perth, doing charter flying in King Air aeroplanes. By charter work I mean, someone might come along with a group of, say, half-a-dozen people and they'd want to go to some place that would take them ages to reach by road, like from Perth to Darwin or Perth to Sydney. So they'd charter an aircraft. It was like a taxi service, really. That's all it was, like an air taxi. Prices varied, of course, and the clients were a mix of tourists and business people, and so pretty soon, I'd done 7500 hours, which included a lot of bush flying.

Then one day in 1968 while I was in Perth I was talking to one of the blokes about flying and he mentioned that the Queensland section of the Royal Flying Doctor Service was advertising for four pilots to replace their previously seconded TAA [Trans-Australia Airlines] pilots. There must've been some sort of change within the organisation there somewhere, and now the RFDS wanted to employ their own pilots.

But I think that my interview for the job deserves some sort of mention. Now, because the senior pilot of TAA was on a trip to Perth, I had a preliminary interview with him to see if I was a suitable applicant for the job with the Flying Doctor Service. That recommendation was positive and it was relayed back to the RFDS Head Office in Brisbane. Then they, the Flying Doctor Service, got in touch and informed me that my final interview was set for ten o'clock, on such-and-such a date, at their Head Office in Queen Street, Brisbane.

Well, that was good news, and so I just assumed that the interview was to be held at ten o'clock in the morning, as you would. But the thing was, I didn't want my employers in Perth to find out that I was going for another job. That just wasn't done in those days, and also my feeling was that there'd be a lot of excellent applicants going for the four RFDS flying jobs. So even though I'd got over the first hurdle and had been recommended, I wasn't all that confident. Anyway, I made up an excuse as to why I couldn't fly for the Perth company on that particular day—the day of my interview in Brisbane—and a friend of mine, who was also a pilot with the same company, he said he'd sub for me, for just that one day.

So, with everything all organised on the Perth workfront, unbeknown to my current employers I flew off to Brisbane for this interview. It didn't cost me anything. The RFDS saw to all that. Accommodation and flights there and back were all paid for.

When I got to Brisbane, I rang the RFDS Head Office to let them know that I'd arrived. 'I'm here,' I said. 'I'll see you tomorrow morning at ten o'clock.'

'Well, no,' they informed me, 'we have interviews already organised throughout tomorrow, sir, and yours isn't set down until ten o'clock tomorrow night.'

Well, that certainly set the cat among the pigeons because I'd only sorted out things back in Perth for that one day. Anyhow, I stayed for my 10 pm interview and caught a flight back to Perth the following day—a day later than expected. So, in saying that it didn't actually cost me anything, well, in a funny sort of way it did, because by the time I returned to Perth the company I was working for had found out that I'd been to an interview for another job. So it was a case of being welcomed back and being told, 'Well, you're finished with us now.'

So, having realised I'd done my last flight with that mob, there followed an extremely nervous wait to see if I'd got the job with the Queensland RFDS. And even though I had all the requirements, including an endorsement on the Queen Air aeroplane, which I'd been flying in Western Australia, as I said, I still wasn't all that confident of getting one of the pilots' positions because I knew there were a lot of very strong applications.

Anyhow, thankfully they gave me the job. That was in May 1968, and my first appointment was out at Charleville, in south-western Queensland. And during the following six or so years I worked at Charleville, I was on call seven days a week, twenty-four hours a day, except for annual holidays. Back then, I'd say that Charleville was the busiest of the RFDS bases. We ran clinics up to four days a week, with overnights at many a remote station property and also at towns like Jundah, Birdsville, Windorah, Thylungra, Bedourie and Thargomindah. On top of all that we then averaged one evacuation per month, to Brisbane.

Then in 1974 I was appointed to the Cairns base, where I worked until my retirement in 1988. So my flying career for the Royal Flying Doctor Service spanned twenty years and, over that time, I clocked up over 20,000 flying hours. But really, because it was my first appointment, the township of Charleville is, and always will remain, very dear to me.

In the Boot

Actually, I got into the Flying Doctor Service in a roundabout sort of way, really. I'd been working out bush as a remote area nurse and the girls from the RFDS knew me and they needed someone to do some relief work for them, so they gave me some relief work and it just followed on from there. I went part-time and finally I went full-time, which was great. That was at our Port Augusta base, which is in South Australia.

Then, as far as stories go, there's one particular accident I still remember quite vividly. It happened to a midwife from Adelaide. At the time she was visiting people on a station property, out along the Trans-continental Railway Line that runs between Port Augusta and Kalgoorlie. I'm not exactly sure how far out the property was just now, but we got an urgent call saying that somehow a brick fence had fallen on this midwife woman and she'd been caught and her lower leg was a mess.

On that occasion we flew out there without a doctor; there was just myself and the pilot. When we landed at the airstrip on the property, there was a ute already waiting for us, so I just grabbed some gear and in we went to see the injured woman. In all, from the time we'd been notified about the accident till the time we arrived, I'd say it took us about an hour and a half to reach her. By then they'd taken the bricks off her and she was lying on the ground, with her foot going in a very odd sort of direction. So I just took one look and I thought, What am I going to do here?

It was a real mess. The pilot even had to walk away from it, that's how horrific it was. Anyhow, the woman was still conscious so I took her pulse and while I was holding her hand I was summing up the situation. What am I going to do? How am I going to go about this?

The wall was a garden wall, and she'd been lying outside on the ground right next to it. Now, I don't know what made it fall over—I didn't actually ever ask that—but when it fell over it pinned her lower leg. It was just like, well, to be absolutely honest, it was a near amputation. Her clothes were even stuck between the broken bones of her leg. Oh, it was sort of all mashed up, mushed up, with the clothes wedged in the break, and I daren't remove them without risking her bleeding more badly than what she already was.

Anyhow, after taking her pulse I thought, well, to start with, I'll cut her shoe off just to see which way her foot's really going. So that's what I did and when I took a look, I thought, there's no way I can reposition this. It's just got to stay in the shape it's in, and I've got to support it the best I can.

Actually, I was a bit worried about not trying to reposition her foot but, anyhow, I ended up deciding to stabilise the fracture as it was, in that awkward position. I put an IV (intravenous drip) in and gave her some pain relief. All this time the people that she'd been staying with were holding up a blanket to give her some shade. It wasn't that hot. It was quite reasonable weather, you know, not too hot or cold, just reasonable. That was a good thing, and I don't remember there being too many flies about either, which was also a very good thing, too. I just hate it when you go to an accident where there's blood and there's millions of flies about.

So I got her as settled as I possibly could and then, when we went to move her back to the aeroplane, we laid her on a mattress—which would've been more comfortable than a stretcher—then we put her in the back of the ute and we drove her back out to the aircraft. To me, that seemed to take about twenty minutes. Then we returned to Port Augusta and from there she was taken down to Adelaide.

And later on I felt justified in my decision not to try and reposition the foot because actually all the doctors and that, they even decided to leave it the way it was before they did the x-rays and everything. They didn't try to do anything until further down the track. And, luckily as it turned out, her leg was saved. Mind you, they had a lot of trouble with it. But they managed to save it, so that was a nice ending to a rather challenging accident.

Then, on a lighter note, there's the story about the same pilot I went out there with on that particular day, when the wall had fallen on the midwife. I won't mention the pilot's name but he was just so funny to work with, which, mind you, is exactly what you need in some of those more serious and critical situations. But this pilot just loved his dog. It went everywhere with him.

Anyway, one time we got this Code One out from Port Augusta. A Code One is an emergency. And when the pilot got the call he just grabbed his gear and ran out of his house. Then, just as he was about to get in his car, he noticed that the boot was open, so he slammed it shut, then he jumped into his car and drove flat out to the airport, where he started preparing the aeroplane for take-off.

Then, just as we're about ready to leave Port Augusta, I get this phone call from his wife saying, 'Rhonda, I can't find his dog anywhere. Is it out there with him?'

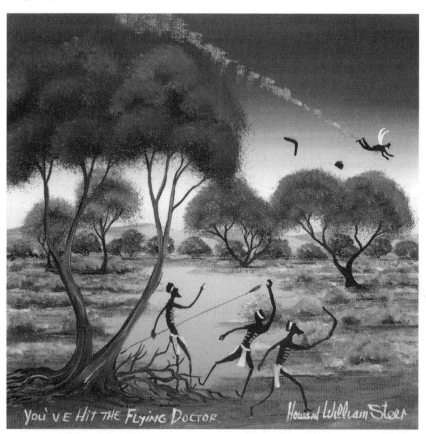

Now, I'd seen the pilot arrive but I hadn't seen his dog.

'No,' I said, 'I haven't seen his dog.'

'Perhaps it's in his car.'

As it happened, I could see his car from where I was and it didn't look like there was a dog in it, so I said, 'No, the dog isn't in the car.'

'Well, that's strange,' his wife said, 'because it always stays around the house when he's gone. Look,' she said, 'just on the off chance, would you mind asking him to check to see if his dog's somehow ended up in the boot of his car?'

So I went out and I told the pilot and sure enough, when he unlocked the boot of his car, there's this sheepish looking dog, looking very pleased to see its even more sheepish looking master.

Injections

I've only ever given injections once and, unless it's a life or death situation, as far as I'm concerned it won't happen again. I just hate giving injections. I don't know why. It's just one of those things. I just can't do it unless, of course, it's an absolute life and death situation. I remember one guy who came in to Gibb River Station, in the Kimberley area of Western Australia. He was up here working in a Main Roads Maintenance Camp, and afterwards he told me that he just knew it was an accident waiting to happen. They apparently had an urn placed out on a bench, with the tap poking outwards so, of course, when he walked past the urn, the tap hooked onto his short pants, didn't it? Over it went and he ended up with boiling water all down his side.

With Gibb River Station being the closest place to where the Main Roads crew were camped, they drove him in and asked if we'd call the Flying Doctor Service and get them to come out and treat him. In the meanwhile, the guy asked for some morphine to ease the pain. Apparently he'd been badly burnt before with a motorbike accident and so this poor bloke he just knew what he was going to have to go through with all these terrible burns. You could actually tell that he was thinking, 'Oh, not again,' if you know what I mean.

Back in those days, the RFDS medical chests contained morphine in both injectable and tablet form; the injections, of course, being the much quicker acting. I mean, we don't have morphine in the medical chests anymore because of the chance of it being abused. But I just couldn't bring myself around to give him an injection, no way, so I gave it to him as a tablet instead. Then, just before the RFDS plane came to pick him up, it came out in discussion that we actually did have morphine in the injectable form. But I just told him that I didn't have the confidence to give him a shot. 'Oh bugger!' he said. 'If I'd known about that I would've given myself the injection!'

Oh, he was a big bikie sort of feller. So it was obvious that it wouldn't have worried him too much to have given himself an injection. But there was no way that I was going to give him one.

Then there was another occasion when I just couldn't give an injection. It's one that really stands out in my mind. It was with a little Aboriginal boy, Devon. He's still around town, here in Derby, but he was only about seven months old when this happened. It was also during the time that my husband and I were out on Gibb River Station.

As usual, these things always seem to happen in the wet season. I don't know why, but the wet's always the worst time for accidents and illness and so forth. Anyhow, Devon's people—his Aboriginal people—came up from Mt Barnett Station and they were all playing cards with our lot at Gibb River Station. Then, as it does quite often in the wet, a huge storm hit us in the afternoon and the house creek just went 'whoosh' and the water level came straight up. We were then flooded in which meant that these Aboriginal people couldn't get back across the house creek to get out to the main road to go home. So they were stranded, and they had this little baby, Devon. He was just there with his grandma and so he wasn't being breastfed or anything. And because they weren't supposed to be staying overnight they hadn't brought along any of the baby formula to feed him with.

Anyhow, they brought this baby, Devon, up to me and asked if I had any baby formula, which we didn't. At that time we didn't even stock baby formula in our store on Gibb River. I tell you, after that we certainly always did. Anyhow, oh, this poor little baby, he was just so sick and I noticed that he had a swollen fontanelle—you know, the little bulging part in his head. Not only that, but he was also very lethargic which to me straight away signified that he could well have had meningitis.

So I got onto the Flying Doctor base in Derby and they suggested that I go to the medical chest and give him an injection. Now, you're supposed to put the injection in the bum, but I just couldn't do it, and especially not to a little baby, no matter how sick he looked. I've seen one of these injections given and, from the reaction, it was really difficult to get the needle into someone, plus it hurt like hell. So you know, I just said to the doctor, 'I'm really, really sorry but no, I can't; not to a little baby like that.' I said, 'I just can't give him an injection. I just can't do it. Is there any other way of treating him?'

Anyhow, we then had to put little Devon on 1000 micrograms of penicillin, as a liquid, which, mind you, is a huge dose of penicillin for a child. But to make matters even worse, with all the rain and the creek having risen so much, the Flying Doctor pilot couldn't land on our strip because it was too wet.

And the Aboriginal people kept saying, 'Why can't they come?'

'They can't come,' I tried to explain, 'because the airstrip needs to dry out before the Flying Doctor aeroplane can land on it.'

'Then why can't they get a chopper (helicopter) to come out for him?'

'They can't,' I said. 'They just can't. It's too overcast for even a chopper to get in.'

Really, there was nothing we could do but sit and wait until the airstrip dried out because, basically, we were stranded. Of course, in the meantime this little fella, Devon, was really struggling. Then I remembered that we had some baby yoghurt in at the clinic and so we fed him with some of this baby yoghurt mixed with water. We also had Sunshine milk but we didn't give him that because it probably would've made him sicker. And dear me, he'd just look at you with this big pair of eyes and your heart just went out to him. He was just so sick, the poor little man.

Then—and my memory's a bit vague here—it was either the next morning or the next afternoon when the RFDS were able to get a plane in. By then the weather had cleared and the house creek had gone down. The house creek does that. It just goes up and down, up and down, like a yo-yo, with each storm, if you know what I mean. But with the Gibb River Station airstrip, it only needs a few hours of sun and it's alright. So they flew in and they got little Devon and they took him in to Derby Hospital, with his grandma.

And Hugh Leslie—who was the RFDS doctor at the time—well, he rang me after and he said, 'Cheryl, you did a really, really good job.' He said, 'He has got meningitis but I think he'll be okay.'

So I felt really proud and very relieved about that, and Devon's nanna also told me, 'Oh, Missus,' she said, 'you shoulda seen him. When they bin' give him that bottle, he bin' like it's all he wanted.'

And that really sticks out in my mind because meningitis is pretty deadly, you know. The poor little fella could've easily died. I really should've given him the needle but you know, again, I just didn't have the confidence. So that's why these days when I see Devon around town I always get a good feeling about that. I guess that he'd probably be about fourteen by now, maybe fifteen.

But there was one old lady who I did give needles to, and that was quite a funny one, in the end really. Old Maggie, it was. She was a beautiful old Aboriginal lady. She used to work in my garden and things like that when we were out on Gibb River Station. And this time she had a terrible dental abscess, so we rang up and we were told that she had to be given one penicillin injection per day, for four straight days.

On the first of the four days, she came into my house and she was nearly as bad as me, so to help her relax I got her to lie down on the bed and I said, 'Wriggle your toes, Maggie. Get ready.'

So she wriggled her toes and I took a deep breath to prepare myself and then one ... two ... three ... and I gave her the first of these daily needles. Anyhow, so that day went okay. We survived it, both Maggie and I. So that was day one. The next day Maggie seemed even more tense, you know, which of course made me feel even worse. So we go through the same procedure; 'Lie down, Maggie. Wriggle your toes,' and I somehow managed to give her the needle. So we both survived day two. Then on the third day Maggie arrives and she's even more tense than the day before and I'm even worse still. She's shaking. I'm shaking. She breaks out in a cold sweat. I'm already in a cold sweat. But we survived the experience ... just. Then come the fourth day she arrives even more tense than the previous three days put together, and by now of course I'm just a complete wreck. Absolute. So I asked her straight out, 'You feel pretty good today, Maggie? You feel okay now?'

And she looked at me with such a look of great relief on her face and she said, 'Yeah, I'm feelin' real good Missus.'

'Good,' I said, 'then how about we won't worry about the needles today, ay, Maggie?'

'Nah, Missus!' she said. 'We don't worry about that no more!'

She didn't want them. I didn't want to give them. And when I told her 'No needles today' she was out of there like a shot. But, oh, they're terrible things to give—just terrible, you know. And that's the only time I've given injections and I don't ever want to give another one again unless, that is, as I said, it's in an absolute life and death situation.

Joe the Rainmaker

Well, it stirs me up a bit just thinking about some of the things I could tell you, especially about the Aboriginal people. But stories like this must be told. They must get out there. Now, don't get me wrong—and I want to make this very clear—this isn't your usual Flying Doctor story. This is not a story like that. In actual fact, the only connection this story has to the RFDS is that it was told to me by two nursing sisters, Brenda Preston and Barbara Struck, who at the time were in charge of the Australian Inland Mission Hospital at Birdsville, up near the South Australian–Queensland border.

Now, I guess you'd know that the Australian Inland Mission [AIM] was the precursor of the Royal Flying Doctor Service in as much as John Flynn was the driving force behind the AIM setting up care facilities and hospitals in remote areas and sending trained nurses out to work in them. Then the Flying Doctor Service was later formed, more or less to support those services of the AIM, plus, of course, any of the other outback support organisations. That's how the RFDS came about.

Anyhow, the AIM Hospital in Birdsville was opened in 1923, and two women by the names of Grace Francis and Catherine Boyd became the first nursing sisters there. It then became their responsibility to provide what was the only community-based health services in that area. And, mind you, it was an area that covered something like 1000 square kilometres. So it was quite vast. What's more, these two women were also responsible for acute first-response emergency care, general outpatients, home and community nursing services, health education and promotion. They also gave advice on public health matters, as well as providing pharmaceutical supplies, basic radiography, administration—the lot—plus they were also, at various times, called upon to provide veterinarian and dental assistance.

Now, my first contact with the actual township of Birdsville didn't happen until much later, in the early 1960s, which by then was when the two nursing sisters, Brenda Preston and Barbara Struck, were in charge of Birdsville's AIM Hospital. At that time I was running the administration for a French mob called the Compagnie Générale de Geophysique, and we were part of a seismic survey party that was constructing a road across the Simpson Desert. That road, or track really, was known as the French Line. Anyhow, Nursing Sisters Preston and Struck became my first port of call for back-up medical support when we were working through that area. So basically I had an office in a caravan out in the desert, and if anybody got sick or was injured I'd take them into the Birdsville Hospital. By that stage, in 1963, the population of Birdsville consisted of eight whites and sixty-three blacks.

Anyhow, I got on very well with these two nursing sisters and they told me some amazing stories, and one of those stories was about an old Aboriginal man called Mintulee, or Joe the Rainmaker as he became known. And I believe that this is a very special story and, like I said, it's one that must be told. But, first, to give you a bit of background. As a young man, Mintulee, as he was originally known, was among just a handful of survivors of an 1888 massacre that was conducted by the Queensland Native Police (QNP). That massacre occurred at a permanent waterhole, at a place called Kaliduwarry, which is on the Eyre Creek. The policeman who organised the massacre was a feller called Sub-Inspector Robert Little and, apparently, what had led to the police attack was the killing of a station cook near Durrie, on the Diamantina River.

Now, that particular massacre by the QNP was timed to wreak the maximum effect on some 200 to 300 young Aborigines who were known to be assembling there at Kaliduwarry. As to just why they were there was that on a regular basis great gatherings of Aboriginal youth were held and these gatherings attracted eighteen-, nineteen- and twenty-year-old Aborigines from as far away as St Vincent Gulf to the south, and the Gulf of Carpentaria to the north. These occasions or gatherings were known as 'Warrthampa ceremonies' and they were held to celebrate the sexual maturity of those Aboriginal youths who were sent to represent their hordes or, as we would call them, tribes. To explain a little further: see, the Aborigines lived in quite small communities that consisted of around thirty people and there were up to eight of those smaller communities within the larger horde. That's how it worked.

But of course to get 200 or 300 natives congregated all together in the one spot provided the perfect opportunity for the Queensland Native Police, because they could just burst in and kill the lot of them. You know, some pastoralist might've simply got in touch and said, 'Hey, they're all gathering out near our place.' So then the QNP came out and of course they were armed with rifles and so forth and so they just went in and, at Kaliduwarry, they hacked to death something like 200 innocent souls. And like so many of these atrocities—and there's no doubting that there have been a great many throughout white history in Australia—the official description of such an event was of it being merely 'a disturbance'. So then it was a case of, 'Oh, wonderful. Job well done, chaps,' and all the records were destroyed.

And I know I'm getting off the track a bit here but to me that's one of the things that us white Australians are really saying 'Sorry' for. It's not simply for just the taking of the Aboriginal children—'the stolen generation', as it's been called. It's also for all the massacres, the murders and the poisonings of the waterholes that have occurred over time. And, believe you me, there are many horrific stories that have been completely blotted out from our history.

Anyhow, that's just some of the background. So this Mintulee, or Joe the Rainmaker as he later became known, and about four or five of his Wangkangurru mates managed to escape the vengeance party at Kaliduwarry that had been led by this Sub-Inspector Robert Little, and they limped back into the desert. The story follows on that a year later Sub-

Inspector Robert Little was said to have fallen from his horse in Birdsville and died of a broken neck. He was subsequently buried in the Birdsville Cemetery—and I'll tell you more about that later at the end of this story.

So then more than ten years passed before Mintulee and what remained of his Wangkangurru horde finally emerged from the southern Simpson Desert to make camp by the Diamantina River, within sight of the township of Birdsville. Like so many of the other native refugees they were attracted by the number of white settlers and their promises of 'keep' in return for work. But of all the Lake Eyre hordes, to the best of my knowledge the Wangkangurru were the last of the Aboriginal peoples to have direct contact with Europeans and, in doing so, they were also the last to relax their own ways in favour of white man's culture. So it must've been a pretty big shock that after all those years of living in freedom, no sooner had Mintulee arrived out of the desert and set up camp by the Diamantina River than he was placed in the care of the local Protector of Aborigines and given a number. Henceforth Mintulee was known by his white protectors simply as 'J11'.

Now, how he then got the name of Joe the Rainmaker was that a feller by the name of George Farwell solemnly declared that Joe had told him how he'd once made the Diamantina come down in flood. And with Birdsville's annual rainfall hovering around the five inch mark—that's if it was lucky— Joe felt duty-bound to relieve all droughts with his well-prepared rainmaking rituals ... in return, of course, for a few shillings for his successes. In her book *From City to the Sandhills of Birdsville*, Mona Henry, who was herself also a Birdsville AIM Nursing Sister from around 1950, actually wrote of Joe's rainmaking requirements, and I quote: 'In bygone days it was human blood, but, in these civilised times, he [Joe the Rainmaker] had to be content with animal blood. Emu feathers, if available, built into a mound over the rainstone, helped bring success to the ceremony. When he was ready he would sing the tribal rainsong and, like Gandhi, was fast to bring results. Rainmakers must be good weather prophets, as I have yet to hear of one dying of starvation. When sufficient rain had fallen, Joe would visit the settlers to collect his fees.'

Anyhow, one time during the early 1960s, when I was visiting Birdsville, Nursing Sisters Preston and Struck went on to tell me about the last days of white treatment for Joe the Rainmaker. By that stage he was quite old—well into his nineties—and even though he was dying in at the AIM Hospital, Joe remained adamant that he wanted to return to his people and await his end, in as natural a manner as possible. But as was the way in those days he was strapped down to his hospital bed for his own good and safety. Then, after he'd been held in his bed for three days, he eventually persuaded the two nurses to release him from the hospital. That they did and so Joe the Rainmaker returned to his camp on the banks of the Diamantina and he positioned himself under a tree, where he could have a good view of everything that was going on. You know, he could see the piccaninnies running around and he was able to see the women going out digging and the men going out hunting and when they'd come back in they'd all see him under the tree.

And the two nursing sisters told me that Joe the Rainmaker survived under that tree for six months. He didn't eat much food and he only asked for water, yet being among his adopted horde and seeing them go about their lives, and being visited constantly by anyone coming and going about the camp, he was kept happy and was fulfilled until the day he died. And isn't that such a great lesson for us more modern-day white Australians, where we tend to stick our aging grandparents or whoever in some God-forsaken nursing home and try to forget about them? Anyhow, as it turned out Joe the Rainmaker ended up living to be ninety-five years of age and he died in the September of 1955.

And here's the nice twist to the story: see, what they did was, when Joe the Rainmaker died, Joe was buried only about a foot away from Queensland Native Police Sub-Inspector Robert Little's grave and in doing so, in silent retribution to the perpetrator of the Kaliduwarry massacre, they laid Joe with his feet on a slight incline towards the head of Little's grave. That's how I first saw their site in 1963, then, a few years later, when I went back to Birdsville, I saw, they'd erected a headstone on Joe's grave and the white cross that had been on Sub-Inspector Robert Little's grave was missing. And that's the story, pretty much as it was told to me by the two Australian Inland Mission nursing sisters, Brenda Preston and Barbara Struck.

Laura

What greatly helped me during my time as a pilot with the Royal Flying Doctor Service in Queensland was the fact that already having been a farmer and earth moving contractor, I could actually relate well to the people on the land and had an appreciation of the demands of their lifestyle. Also what came in very handy was my many years of remote area flying, and that gave me the experience and ability to access the roads, paddocks, clay flats and bush strips, with regard to the capabilities of both the aircraft and myself, as a pilot.

That being said, flying still threw up many challenges, especially before the introduction of GPS [Global Positioning System]. One such case occurred at Laura, a small remote Cape York location west of Cooktown. Laura held a number of festivals, the two major ones being the Laura Festival, which was a big indigenous dance festival, and then there was the local Laura Races. And of course from time to time there would be a few flare-ups, or altercations, at these festivals, which meant that medical attention or even an evacuation was required.

There was one time I remember being called to Laura on a very wet and foggy night to evacuate a local who was thought to have broken his neck in a horse accident. I flew out there with a female doctor and on our arrival Laura was shrouded in stratus cloud. So, with severely limited visibility, before coming below lowest safe altitude I got in contact with Percy Trezise. Percy was a local identity and I knew that he'd flown his own aircraft to Laura to attend that particular festival. He was a former TAA captain who by this time had done a lot of flying throughout Cape York. Now, because I knew that Percy had his aircraft at Laura, I wanted to speak to him on the radio and ask him if he'd let me know when I was over the top of the strip.

Anyhow, I got in radio contact with Percy and while I was getting directions I circled for about fifteen minutes without being able to see anything. Not a thing. All the while, the female doctor on board had the headphones on and so she was listening in on our conversation. And because of the tone of Percy and my discussion, plus our obvious lack of visibility, I think the poor doctor might've started to get a bit concerned about the situation, because at one stage she decided that just maybe the patient didn't have a broken neck after all and perhaps the evacuation could wait until the following morning!

Still, I'd been to Laura hundreds of times before and, knowing the area as well as I did, I assured the doctor not to worry because, with Percy's help, I felt confident of being able to carry out a safe landing. Now, I'm not sure if she was all that convinced about my ability but I went ahead anyway and carried out a let-down safely in heavy cloud. I then advised Percy that when I thought I was on final approach I'd put on my landing lights and he could inform me as to exactly where I was in relation to the airstrip. I then continued descent and, much to the relief of the doctor, all went according to plan. With Percy's help we had no trouble landing and, later on, the take-off to evacuate the injured person also went without a problem.

Now, while we're talking about the festivals out at Laura, another sort of funny thing happened. On an earlier occasion we'd been called out there at night to evacuate Cecil, an Aboriginal employee of Susan and Tom Shepherd. Susan and Tom were from Artemis Station. Cecil had gone off to the festival and had, unfortunately for him, got into a 'blue'—a fight—and his stomach had been cut open quite badly with a broken bottle. We'd been advised that there was—and I quote—'already a doctor on the scene'. Apparently this doctor had been attending the festival and we were assured that he'd look after Cecil until our arrival.

So we flew out there to Laura. The only trouble was that when we arrived it turned out that the doctor who we'd been assured was already on the scene, looking after Cecil, was actually an eye specialist, who I attended regularly. Of course, this injury of Cecil's was a little out of the ordinary to what he usually dealt with on a daily basis. So I think the eye specialist was just as glad as poor old Cecil was to hear the throb of our noisy engines in the distance. And all went well with our landing and take-off on that occasion.

But another time when I had a bit of a mix-up was during an election and, naturally, the people of Cape York

Peninsula had to make sure they exercised their right to vote, along with the rest of us. To that end Susan Shepherd loaded up her ute with people from her property to go into Laura for voting day. The trip in went without incident and everyone cast their vote. But then on their return journey an altercation occurred between one of the indigenous women and her bloke. I'm not sure what it was about, whether it was of a personal or political nature, but without thinking of the consequences, mid-altercation, this woman simply picked up her port—suitcase—and stepped off the back of the ute.

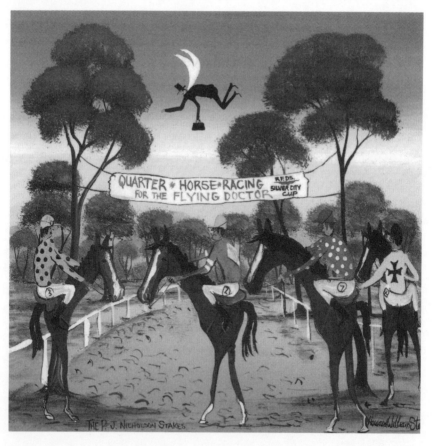

Now, unfortunately, the ute was travelling along at over sixty kilometres per hour and so the woman suffered quite severe head injuries.

Anyhow, that night I received a call from the RFDS doctor to say we were needed to evacuate this injured woman from Kimba Station—Kimba being the nearest station to where the accident had occurred. So we took off in the Queen Air and headed out to Kimba. Being set among thick scrub as it was, I knew Kimba Station would be difficult to locate, especially at night. But, as was standard practice, I was fully expecting to be guided to the remote property by some car lights lining the strip, awaiting our arrival.

On this occasion, for some reason or other that I've forgotten, that didn't happen. I couldn't see anything at all. But then after flying around for a while in the dark I finally saw some lights on the ground and so I headed in that direction. When I arrived over the property, there were still no car lights to greet me so, by using the Queen Air's landing lights, I picked out the strip near the house and landed there safely. A vehicle soon arrived on the scene and out popped a very surprised family. I looked at them. They looked at me.

'This isn't Kimba Station, is it?' I said.

'No,' came the reply. 'This is Violet Vale Station.'

Anyhow, they were able to give me directions and about half an hour later we landed safely at Kimba Station and the evacuation took place without further confusion.

Lombadina

Back in the 1980s I was working in a voluntary capacity, up in the Kimberley region in the far north of Western Australia. If you know that area, I worked for about four years at Lombadina Aboriginal Mission. I also worked for a year in Derby. Following that I spent a year up at the Kalumburu Aboriginal Mission. Then I worked for another year in what was originally known as Port Keats, which is now known as the Wadeye Aboriginal Community. And with the Royal Flying Doctor Service having a base at Derby, most weeks they used to fly out to all those places to run medical clinics plus, at the drop of a hat and normally at night—and usually in the worst of weather conditions—they'd fly in for emergency 'medi-air-vacs', as we called them.

So yes, you could say I've had some 'interesting' times at some of those Aboriginal communities that have been linked in with the RFDS. Take Lombadina for example; I think there were about 200 people there in the mid-1980s. Back then, they had a pressed gravel airstrip, made up to a certain standard, which was similar to most of those other places I worked at in the Kimberleys. Lombadina had a generator as well, though from memory, I don't think it had the capacity to be able to light up the airstrip. Anyway, the generator was too far away from the airstrip to run the necessary electrical lines or what have you.

So of course when there's a night emergency, first of all there's the having to go out in the middle of the night—and, as I said, it was usually in the most atrocious of weather conditions—and sort out the kerosene lamps to light the strip for the plane to come in and out. The kero lamps were built like a large double cone, with a big reservoir of kero and a wick on the top. They had a good, big light but their only problem was that they lacked any decent wind protection. So if it was too windy or, you know, if it was too wet and stormy to light the kero lamps, which happened a lot up there, you had to con all the blokes into getting out there in their four-wheel drives to line up alongside the airstrip.

For the plane to land safely, you lined the cars up at a good distance apart and they'd be pointing alternately across the airstrip so that their lights weren't aimed at each other. You could say that they were sort of like in a zigzag formation and then you had one or two vehicles right down the very end, on low beam, so that the pilot could gauge where the end of the strip was. And of course there were other things to sort out like always having to clear the cattle off the airstrip. They were a particular danger, especially at Lombadina. We had free range cattle up there and so we had to make sure they didn't get in the way of the plane. So that was all good fun, though I suppose everyone's heard all those type of stories.

With Lombadina, I don't know what the legals were, but away back when the Sacred Heart Nuns and St John of God were the mainstays of the missions, the original people up on the Dampier Peninsula—the Bard Tribe—gave the land to the Church. In those early days the place was just about self-sufficient; you know, for meat, bread, vegetables and so forth. So there wasn't too much they had to bring in, other than fuel and things like that. Then over time the particular religious orders gave the Aborigines the leasing rights to the land, plus the cattle, plus all the windmills and the stockyards that were dotted around the place. We ran the vegetable gardens and the bakeries and the mechanical workshops and all those sort of self-functioning things that were needed to keep the place going. Then over time the Aborigines also took over those functions. Take the bakery, for instance; rather than ship bread up from Broome they had someone baking the mission bread in a nice wood-fired oven and when I ran the store I sold that bread in the store on a commission basis. That's how it worked.

Of course the Aborigines were very itinerant. Sometimes they lived in Broome, sometimes they'd come back out to the mission at Lombadina or they might even go and live more traditionally out on their original beach locations and things like that. And other than the usual weekly clinic duties that the RFDS ran, some of the sort of emergency casualties we'd have were things like childbirths, general accidents and injuries and—you know, I shouldn't say it—but there were the injuries from fights and things like that which was usually the result of some alcohol-related dispute or the like.

But the traditional mourning ceremonies were something very interesting. Different cultures might do it a different way but, with the Bard people, the way they did it up there was that they had what was called a 'smoking ceremony'. Now, I'm not an Aboriginal anthropologist or anything so you'll have to check the facts on this, but it was all to do with smoking the spirits away or as a cleansing process to release the spirits out of the body. And sometimes there were lots of little fires made from gum leaves that were set around the coffin and at other times they carried the coffin past a big fire and the winds blew the smoke across it. Then, you know, because it was a Christian Mission, after the smoking ceremony ninety percent would then have a Catholic Mass in the Church followed by a normal Christian burial, which was held in the cemetery just right behind the church.

I remember one extremely moving 'smoking' they held was when they brought back the body of one of the old-time Aborigines to Lombadina. It was one of the old male Elders. They flew in at night for that one and so we had to light up the airstrip. The old man had died and I think the RFDS took the body to Derby for an autopsy, or for some sort of legal thing, then they brought him back for their traditional mourning ceremony, which was this 'smoking'.

So the RFDS plane landed at night and the Aboriginal people came up and they took the body—the coffin—out of the plane and I think they took it back to the house of one of the Elders' relatives. The coffin was still closed, and they had a mourning ceremony with those people and that's when they had the smoking ceremony. Then after that they had the traditional Christian Mass and burial. That was quite a big one, that was. Well, I know I've gone off the track a little but really what I'm trying to get across is that the Royal Flying Doctor Service was a very strong link up there, all throughout the Kimberley region in so many and varied ways. So yes, they are a great organisation and, personally, for me, the time I spent up there was an unreal yet a really great experience.

Long Days, Great Times

You could just about title this story 'The Longest Day', because to begin with the Royal Flying Doctor Service Base in Alice Springs rang me at home at two o'clock in the morning and said, 'We've had an accident case up at Tennant Creek. It's pretty serious so could you fly up there and bring them back down to the Alice?'

In those days, Tennant Creek only had one doctor, and a few nurses and I knew that the surgeon was in Alice Springs. So I said, 'Yeah, no problem.'

So we jumped in the De Havilland Dove and I took off at about three o'clock in the morning and we headed off to Tennant Creek. I'd say that it would've taken us about two hours to fly up there, then we spent about half an hour on the ground, then two hours back—which is four hours' flying time—so I guess that would've had us back in the Alice at around seven thirty.

We also had a short routine medical visit scheduled for that day. That was supposed to finish at about midday or one o'clock. Now, you don't like to change those if you can help it, because at these remote stations and settlements everyone comes into town especially to see us. So after we got back from Tennant Creek I said, 'Look, let's still do the routine medical visit.'

Okay, so we did the medical visit, then we'd just got back in to Alice Springs when the hospital rang up and said, 'Do you feel like flying back to Tennant Creek? We've got a real serious case of peritonitis.'

From memory the appendix had burst and one thing had led to another and things didn't look too good, so I said, 'Yeah. Right-o, no problem. I'll go back to Tennant Creek.'

So I flew to Tennant Creek for the second time that day and I'd just arrived home again when the phone rang. It was the surgeon in Alice Springs—I knew him quite well—and he said, 'Neil, they tell me you've already had a bugger of a day. Well, I'm having a bugger of a day, too. I've got this woman here but the longer we keep her on the anaesthetic machine, the more chance she's got of getting brain damage.' He said, 'Look, I've done everything I can possibly do up here and I'd really like to get her down to Adelaide straightaway.'

As it happened, I was the only pilot up in Alice Springs at that time who could do the trip because the De Havilland Dove was an IFR [Instrument Flight Rules] aircraft and I was the only instrument rated pilot around the place. So it had to be me. 'Right-o,' I said. 'Yeah, we'll go.'

As soon as that decision had been made, they then had to make enough space in the Dove to fit in the anaesthetic machine. And so, while I was flight planning, the engineer was busy stripping the seats out of the aircraft so that we could fit the anaesthetic machine and everything else in. I'd say that the machine itself must've been about eight or nine feet long and about three feet wide so it only just barely squeezed in the door. Then I also wanted to scrape every ounce of fuel we could get into the tanks, and so they were filled to the absolute. Actually, in the end we were a little bit overloaded, but I don't think I even bothered with a load sheet.

Anyhow, so then I took off for Adelaide. By that time it was probably about eight or nine o'clock at night. On board with me were the female patient of course, plus a doctor and a nursing sister. But because we didn't have 240 volt power, the doctor and nurse had to work the anaesthetic machine manually. They had to do all the pumping and everything. And on that trip I was in cloud the whole time. I didn't even see a star. Not a single one. It was pitch black. I never even saw a single light on the ground or anything. And normally when you'd go on a long trip like that, the nursing sisters had a big flask of coffee or something to help you keep alert. But that wasn't the case on this occasion. They were so flat out in the back, caring for the patient and doing the pumping and so forth, that they didn't even get the chance to come up and chat with me. So the only thing that kept my sanity was talking on the radio and watching the DME [Distance Measuring Equipment] tick over.

Anyhow, as you might be able to imagine, I was pretty stuffed by the time we finally began our descent into Adelaide. And when we broke out of the cloud, at about 500 feet, it was as clear as a bell. And with seeing the lights of Adelaide and then there ahead, less than a mile in front of me, was the runway, oh gees, I tell you, Adelaide was the most beautiful sight I'd ever seen. And I still reckon it's the prettiest thing I've ever seen because, as I said, for five hours I hadn't seen a thing outside the cockpit, not even a star. Nothing.

Then by the time we landed at Adelaide I worked out that I'd spent eighteen hours in the air and that's not including the time on the ground. But you see back then, there was no one else in Alice Springs who was qualified to fly on instruments apart from me. So that was my longest day: eighteen stick hours in one day. And except for long-distance flights, I'd say that that record would never be broken because these days, first, there's always plenty of properly trained pilots available and second, there's usually plenty of available aircraft around.

Anyway, the woman survived, and I guess that's the most important thing.

So yes, Alice Springs was an extremely fascinating part of my life. Plus it's also what you make it, isn't it? Because, you know, you can go on about the aircraft and one thing and another and, I mean, of course, we didn't have all this fancy stuff they've got today. We even took the auto-pilot out of the aircraft because it weighed too much. The damn thing usually never worked anyway. But, see, originally up in Alice Springs we just had the one doctor, the one sister, the one pilot, the one aircraft and the one engineer. Then over the years the medical side of it built up to such an extent that when I left they replaced me with two pilots and two aircraft. By then I'd flown 1812 hours in three years. That's 600 actual flying hours per year, and for that sort of work you'd normally expect to fly a maximum of about 400 hours a year. But that's what used to happen in those early days and that's why they doubled up the service after I left.

And with us just having the one engineer, the one pilot and the one aircraft, we still kept our aircraft virtually as good as new. I'd write the most minute snags on a piece of paper and stick it on the wall in the engineer's office and he'd fix them up. We had that aircraft in absolutely 'Mickey Mouse' condition. Actually, the whole time I was there I only ever broke down once, and that had nothing to do with our own engineer. It was because of some sort of a fault in overhaul maintenance while it was in Sydney. What happened was that the aircraft had its usual two-yearly major service in Bankstown and when they put the fuel line on they were supposed to use two spanners on it. But they only used the one spanner and they twisted the fuel line and in doing so they twisted the pipe.

Then after the plane came back from being serviced I went out to a property one day and everything seemed to be going well. But then on our way back home I got up to about 8000 or 9000 feet and the fuel pressure started dropping off and the engine began surging. So I shut the engine down. And that's what they found out afterwards—that the pipe had twisted causing a drop in pressure and, at the high ambient temperature, the fuel vapourised. It was just something as simple as that.

Anyway, after I shut the engine down I said to the doctor, 'Well,' I said. 'Here we are, we're on one engine and it's about two hundred miles to Alice Springs. That's a bit too far to go on just the one engine.'

I mean, I could've had a go at it but you don't push your luck in an aeroplane. Never. So then I had to find the closest suitable airstrip to land on the one engine and so we went back to Ernabella Mission. I'm not sure what it's like now but back then Ernabella was a dry mission. Even the merest mention of alcohol there was frowned upon. So we were then stuck at Ernabella Mission for two days without a drink.

Anyway, in those days Alice Springs had a population of only about 3000 or 4000 people, and word gets around. So by the time we got back, everyone knew that we'd been stuck out on a dry settlement at Ernabella. Then the instant we walked into the Memorial Club the barmaid plonked these two huge pots of beer down in front of us. We didn't have to say a thing. And that's what the people were like out there in the Alice. Absolutely great. They knew where we'd been and they reckoned we'd be in need of a big beer so they got the barmaid to pour us one as soon as we walked in the club. So yes, we might've had some long days but, gee, they were great times.

Looked like Hell

My name is now Clemson, though O'Connor was my maiden name when I was working as an emergency flight nurse for the Royal Flying Doctor Service, out in the west of New South Wales, at both Broken Hill and Dubbo. These days I'm married and we're living on a property just outside Walgett, in the central-north of NSW. But I was with the Flying Doctor Service for nine years and I enjoyed every moment of it ... well, almost ... because during my time with the RFDS we had to deal with many and varied incidents. Some you could draw humour from. Some were tough to take. So it was not always easy, no.

Now I know that tragic stories don't make for the best of reading but I do remember one time at Moomba, up in the north-eastern corner of South Australia. The Flying Doctor Service had the contract at the Moomba oil and gas fields so we used to go out there and it was absolutely amazing—the harshness of the place and just how unbelievably hot it can get. And this story really brings that sort of thing home to you.

Anyhow, they had a bloke out there who was new to the job so he wasn't acclimatised and so he was unaware of the damage that that sort of scorching heat can do to you. Now, I can't remember what his actual job was but he was working about a hundred foot up in the air, doing something on one of those big rigs they've got, and he was out in the sun for about three hours without drinking enough water. So it was purely dehydration that got him because someone just happened to look up and there he was, hanging upside-down in a safety harness, swinging in midair and he was fitting [having a fit].

That's when we got the call to fly out and get him. In the meantime, the nurses that were based up at Moomba, they had to somehow get up this big rig and they had to go out to where he was hanging to get the drip into him and then get him down. It was just from him purely being overcooked. And actually he was very lucky to even be alive because his whole body had virtually collapsed. He had muscle meltdown. His kidneys were shutting down. He was bleeding from absolutely every orifice. Everything. Then when we arrived we had to ventilate him, and it was difficult because we couldn't see for all the blood that was pouring out of him from everywhere. In all, it took probably eight hours to stabilise him.

So we flew him down to Adelaide and when we got there we got him into the ambulance and we had an emergency police escort from the airport into Royal Adelaide Hospital. Oh, we had all the lights flashing and all the sirens blaring— everything. They even shut the traffic lights off so that we could get him to the hospital quicker. Then, when we got to the hospital, all the lifts were opened for us, and I think they worked on him for another three or four hours. After that he had to be put on dialysis and then he was on ventilators for a long time.

Looked like Hell

And now he's back at Moomba. He's just doing light duties, mind you. He might still have a few problems but he's a very lucky man to still be alive, with what he went through. So that was a very difficult one, particularly for the nurses at Moomba who had to get right out of their comfort zone and get up the rig and treat the man while he was hanging upside-down and fitting in midair. I mean, you really have to admire people with a commitment like that, don't you?

Then there's another story. This one's also about someone who had to get out of their comfort zone to help a patient, though in a different sort of way. Actually, I'm reminded of this story because just last night we had a storm out here at Walgett. We only had about forty points or something but it was bad enough to cut the power and cut the road. Mind you, the rain's nice and welcome, that's for sure.

But talking about rain reminds me of the time when I was working for the RFDS in Broken Hill and a woman rang us from a property up near the Queensland border. In this case this woman had very little medical knowledge. Apparently they'd had a lot of rain up there and her husband had been out riding his motorbike and it had slipped from underneath him and he'd fallen off, damaging his leg. Unfortunately, they only had a dirt airstrip on their property so we couldn't fly in there at the time, because it was too wet. So we then had to try and instruct the husband's wife, over the telephone, as to what to do and how to go about it.

As I said this woman had very limited medical knowledge but from her description of the injuries her husband had obviously broken the leg, and the break was both the tibia and fibula; yes, both of them. In fact, it was a compound fracture, meaning that bone was sticking out which, as you might be able to imagine, was causing the husband a lot of pain and the woman a lot of anxiety.

So, first we had to treat the pain. For that the woman had to give her husband an injection of pethidine, which was kept in the RFDS medical chest. The only trouble was that she'd never given a needle before. Oh, I think perhaps she might've given a few jabs to some of their cattle or something which, mind you, as it turned out, proved to be a very good training ground. So initially we instructed her how to give the injection for the pain, and she managed that.

The next problem was that, from what she'd told us, it was obvious that the foot wasn't getting enough blood to it. She described the foot as being 'cold and white'. Of course, we didn't want to lose the foot, so after her husband had settled down a bit from the pethidine we had to reduce the fracture in an attempt to keep up the blood flow. Now, to reduce the fracture, the woman had to manually— physically—put the bone back into alignment. And she had to do it all by herself, and unpractised, because there was nobody out there to help her. There was just her and her husband. The only help she had was us, and we were miles away on the end of a telephone.

So we told her how to manipulate the bone back into alignment, which is done by pulling and pulling, as hard as she could, until the bone pops back into place. Naturally, she was a bit apprehensive at first but, with the fate of her husband's foot in the balance, she eventually gathered up the courage and in fact, as it turned out, she managed to do that quite well too. So she got the bone back into alignment and then, because she didn't plaster it or anything like that, she had to keep the leg elevated by putting it on a pillow. Once that was done it was important to keep the husband resting. Then throughout the night she had to keep checking for the pulse, just to make sure that blood was still getting down into the foot. All during this time she was in constant contact with us.

Of course, before we could get the aeroplane in there to pick up her husband and get him back to the Broken Hill Hospital, we had to wait until the airstrip was safe enough for us to land. As it happened, they didn't get any more rain that night and so things looked promising. So the next morning she had to somehow get her husband out of the house and into a vehicle and then drive out and check the condition of the airstrip. She also had to clear the kangaroos from off the strip and check for any holes and twigs or sticks or logs that might get in our way.

Anyhow, after she gave us the all-clear, we flew in there. By then it was about twenty-four hours after the accident. And the woman had done a great job. The leg was looking really good and her husband was relatively pain free. The only trouble was, it'd obviously been a very long and harrowing ordeal for the woman because she looked like absolute hell.

Looking at the Stars

If you like, first of all I've got a story here that's a little bit humorous. It's one that, these days, has almost become part of Flying Doctor Service folklore because you'll hear it, or differing versions of it, being told in just about every pub around western Queensland. What's more, it's a true story. That's what I've been told, anyway.

Now, I haven't got an exact date but at one time the Charleville base of the RFDS received a call from a ringer, and the ringer said, 'Doc, yer gotta come real quick. Me mate's hurt his hand real bad.'

Anyhow, in an attempt to find out how the accident happened, and to get a clearer idea as to just how badly the ringer's mate's hand was damaged, the doctor tried to extract a little bit more information out of the ringer. But, with ringers being ringers and ringers, more often than not, being men of extremely few words, the doctor couldn't get much more information out of him other than his mate had 'hurt his hand real bad' and that the doctor had better 'come real quick'.

So they jumped into the plane and off they went. After they landed at the particular station property where the accident had occurred, they rushed to the scene and there was this ringer, the one with the damaged hand, sitting there looking sad and sorry and forlorn and the other ringers were sort of sheepishly standing around behind him. Anyhow, the doctor walked up to the injured ringer and said, 'Show me your hand, son.'

Which he did. He lifted his hand up and his thumb was totally missing. It was gone.

'Where's your thumb?' the doctor asked.

Well, the injured ringer, who was also a man of few words, didn't say anything but simply motioned towards his mates. So the doctor said to his mates, 'Where's his thumb? What've you done with his thumb?'

'Oh,' one of them said, 'we stuck it over there, on the gatepost, fer safe keepin'.'

And just as doctor turned around to the gatepost, he saw a crow heading skyward, thumb and all. So I don't know how the ringer had actually lost his thumb in the first place, but it had certainly gone missing after the crow had flown off with it.

So that's one story. But I suppose that every time I go out to the bush I come back with another story and this one came about when we were putting together a promotional DVD for the Royal Flying Doctor Service. There was just myself, the director and a cameraman, and we'd based ourselves at Mount Isa and we were filming right up to Bentinck and Sweers Islands. Bentinck and Sweers Islands are just off Burketown, into the Gulf of Carpentaria.

But where this story actually comes from is Burketown itself, and I thought it was rather beautiful. The lady that looks after the Burketown Clinic—if you like, she's the registered nurse there—her name is Glenda. She's an Aborigine, and we fly in there once a week and conduct a clinic. Now Burketown, as you may well know, is a very remote location. Just check it up on your map.

So we were there filming in Burketown and the director happened to ask Glenda, 'Seeing that you're the only one with any form of medical expertise out here in this remoteness, in a situation of an accident of a night time, how do you handle it all on your own?'

And Glenda said to the director, 'Well, first I patch them up as best I can. Next, I call the Flying Doctor and then I go out to the airstrip and I look up at the stars and just wait for one to get bigger.'

Memories of Alice Springs

When John Flynn died in 1951, my father, Fred McKay, took over his position of Superintendent of the Australian Inland Mission. When that happened we moved from Brisbane down to Sydney. Then we'd only been in Sydney for about a year or so and there were some financial problems or other within the organisation of the AIM. I was a bit too young to know all the details about it but it's been well documented. Anyhow, in amongst all that, they were having problems getting staff for the AIM's Bush Mother's Hostel, up in Alice Springs. So my mother, Meg McKay, volunteered her services to be Matron—gratis—and so we all moved up to Alice Springs. By all, I mean it was really just my mother, my elder sister, my brother and myself because Dad still had all his other AIM duties to attend to, so he was coming and going a lot.

The Bush Mother's Hostel was in Adelaide House. That's in Todd Street. It's a National Trust building now, like a museum. And I guess that you know all about how John Flynn actually helped redesign the hostel, with the wide verandahs and the natural sort of air conditioning. That was where the air came up from a tunnel under the building, to cool the place down. I would've only been twelve or so, at that stage, but back then Alice Springs was quite a small town. I'd say that there would've only been about two or three thousand people. They'd just built their first high school, the year before we went up there and so I was in the first group of students to go to that new high school.

But it was a fascinating place and it just seemed to me that Alice Springs encapsulated a great range of people—people who were all unique, in their own sorts of ways. You know, everyone seemed to be a character who lived their character. And there's books out now about some of these people where they're described as being 'outback heroes and outback identities'.

One lady in particular comes to mind. Her name was Olive Pink. At that time I didn't have a clue as to what Olive did but you'd always see her looking like she was someone out of Edwardian England. Wherever she went, she wore these long white dresses, with a white hat and a white scarf, and gloves. And in a place like Alice Springs that was very much a look that was out of place. But, as I said, while I was there I didn't know what she did and since then I've learned that she was a quite well known conservationist and environmentalist. Apparently she was very instrumental in opening up and saving a lot of the native vegetation throughout that area. There's even the Olive Pink Memorial Gardens there now and I believe she helped establish a lot of that garden herself. But when you're only in your early teenage years ... well, my memories of her were just of seeing her around town and thinking what a strange lady she was.

Then when they started to build the John Flynn church, Dad was back a lot more because he was supervising the building. So we watched the John Flynn church being built. And if you're ever up that way, it's well worth a visit, not only because of its basic structure, but there's also a lot of symbolism in the actual building, which is something that a lot of people don't realise. It's set out like a story of the life of John Flynn and his achievements.

Anyway, I always thought it was just interesting, how some of the things Dad did in Alice Springs seemed to have had far-reaching effects for different people. There was another fellow called Ted Smith. Ted didn't have any work but he owned a truck. He was married with two kids. So he was struggling to make a go of things. Then, in the early days of getting the church under way, he sort of turned up one day and offered Dad any help he could give. Of course, back then everything was being shipped up from Adelaide. But just at that point in time there was some sort of big transport problem or other and this Ted Smith arrived just at the right time, with this truck, and saved Dad a momentous problem. And that set Ted Smith up in Alice Springs. He helped Dad out with the building of the church, then he went on to become a very, very highly respected businessman who had this very prolific business, not only in transport but I think he also diversified into other areas.

But us kids, we thought that the whole thing was all just one big adventure because there were times when we'd go out from Alice Springs on different trips with Dad, and we'd camp out on the ground, with the flies and the mosquitoes and everything else, and that was just an accepted part of our lives.

And talking about going out camping and some of the people of Alice Springs; something that always amazed me was that while Dad was overseeing the building of the John Flynn church he was always looking for local materials to build it with. Anyhow, there's quite a bit of a special type of pink marble in the church, and I remember going out in the truck with Dad one time and he'd especially asked these two old Aboriginal fellows to come out and help him find some of this pink marble. So there we were, driving around, away out in the middle of nowhere, north of Alice Springs somewhere, and all of a sudden these old Aborigines told Dad to stop. So he did, and they pointed to a place.

'Over there,' they said.

To me, all the rocks looked exactly the same. But when we took a closer look, there it was. And you would have never known that there was pink marble there until you'd started chipping away at the rock. But somehow ... and don't ask me how ... they just knew it was there.

News Flash

You know, I've been involved in a lot of things up in the gas fields at Moomba and, actually there's not too many funny stories that come out of there. Tragedies aren't good for a book but here's one that has a lighter side to it. It's all hooked into the Flying Doctor Service, and it's probably a case where we did people more of a dis-service than a service, though, it was a sort of humorous dis-service.

I hadn't been at Moomba all that long and what happened was that in about the early 1990s, up in the far north of South Australia, it was one of those very rare times when Lake Eyre was flooded, okay. And when Lake Eyre floods a lot of tourists like to go out there and have a look because it's such an amazing sight, what with all the wildlife and that. Anyhow, all these tourist people, to get a closer look, what they do is they charter aeroplane flights out from places like William Creek or Port Augusta or Leigh Creek and they go out and fly over the lake.

Now, I don't know if you've ever seen Lake Eyre in flood but it's a fantastic experience. And what happens is that when it floods, in most places it's still only got about two foot of water in it, and because it's so salty, on a really calm day when you fly over the lake, it's like flying over a mirror. It's like an optical illusion. You could be flying at a hundred feet and you look down and it seems like you're at 30,000 feet, and if you've got clouds above you, you'll also get that cloud reflection off Lake Eyre. It's quite phenomenal.

The other thing that's unusual about Lake Eyre is that it's below sea level, right, so when you're flying a plane over it, it's difficult to gauge exactly how high you are. Because in a case like that, when the aeroplane's altimeter tells you that you're at true ground level, you could actually be something like a hundred feet off the ground. Add to that the mirror imagery that I was talking about and you'll understand why most pilots are a bit wary about flying too low over Lake Eyre.

So, now to the story. There was one particular charter flight full of oldies—what you'd call 'snow birds'—and the charter pilot took these snow birds over the lake and of course they all wanted to have a real good, close, look. The pilot, for whatever reason, mustn't have been paying too much attention as to how high the plane was off the deck and he got a bit low and he ploughed right into the middle of Lake Eyre. Fortunately nobody was hurt, apart from the pilot's ego getting bruised, that is. Anyway, the plane sort of bounced along the water and—'chung'—it ground to a halt. Then what happened was that the plane's emergency global positioning alert system went off and that's when we were asked to go and do a search-and-rescue to look for this plane. As soon as we got the story we thought, 'Okay, it's highly likely that it's one of those scenic flights, you know, over Lake Eyre.'

Anyway, we take off in the helicopter and we fly out to Lake Eyre. Now, after the plane had come to a stop, all these snow birds had managed to get themselves out of the plane. As I said, nobody was hurt but they were all very wet, you see, and it was a pretty cold day with a bit of wind, so they were cold and wet and miserable. So these oldies, they came up with an idea to help increase their chances of being found and so they took most of their wet clothes off and they placed them down on the wing of the plane in such a way that they wrote the word 'HELP'. That not only let anyone flying

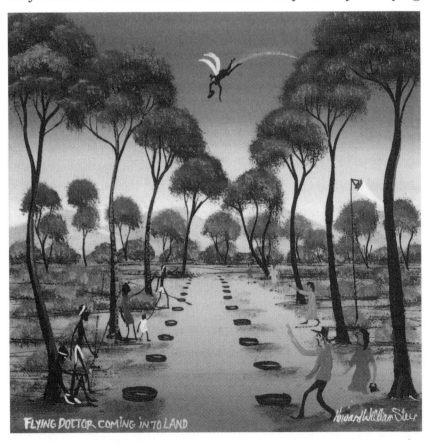

FLYING DOCTOR COMING INTO LAND

overhead know that they were in trouble but it also helped to dry their clothes out, you see.

So we picked up the signal—the emergency alarm—on the helicopter and we sort of tracked them by the signal until we saw them. They were just this dot in the middle of Lake Eyre. Then the helicopter pilot said, 'Look, I can't land in water.' So he said, 'We'll fly over to reassure them that we know where they are and then we'll head to the nearest station property and sort things out from there.'

'Righto,' I said. 'No worries.'

So we flew in on the helicopter and this's where we did these poor old snow birds a bit of a dis-service, right. We flew in on the helicopter, nice and close until we could see that they were waving at us and they could see that we were waving back. We just wanted to reassure them that they'd been seen. But then, as we pulled away in the helicopter, we created this huge updraft and the updraft just lifted all their clothes up in the air and scattered them back into the water. So their clothes had almost dried but now they're all wet again. And they weren't too happy about it either because they're now shaking their fists at us, the poor buggers.

Anyhow, we contacted the people at the nearest station, which was Muloorina Station, just on the edge on Lake Eyre, and when we arrived there they had some flat bottom boats; they're like punts. So we basically got some four-wheel drives and we got as close to the ditched aeroplane as we could, which was about probably two or three kilometres. Then we put these flat bottom boats in the water and we sort of walked them out to the aeroplane. Then we piled all these cold, wet and miserable snow birds into these boats and then we walked them back in relays to the shore. From there we got them in the four-wheel drives and took them back to Muloorina Station. Then, the next day, a couple of planes flew in to pick them all up.

But the odd thing about it was, when we first went to Muloorina Station to sort out how we were going to rescue the snow birds, two aeroplanes landed almost simultaneously. One was the RFDS plane from Port Augusta, who'd been asked to come up just in case we needed back-up, and right behind that was the Channel 9 news plane from Adelaide. Now, how on earth they found out about the accident so fast, I would not have a clue.

But anyway, the Channel 9 plane landed and it was really funny because, here we are, out on an outback station, you know, and it'd been a bit of a tough day, so everybody's a bit rough around the gills and looking tardy and the lady from the Channel 9 news crew steps out of their plane, and she's immaculately dressed. Perfect. She looked like she'd just walked right out of a page of a fashion magazine. She'd put her lippy on and changed her dress and everything and then she started running around wanting to interview everybody. And, you know, we're saying, 'Look, excuse me, can't you see that we're a little bit busy trying to co-ordinate a rescue here?'

But it astounded me just how quickly the news crew flew up from Adelaide, to land at this station in an attempt to get the story. But in the end the news people turned out to be okay, really. You know, we were all still there at last light, and after they'd got their story they stayed on at the station with the rest of us, and we all bunked down in the shearers' quarters together, and then they let their hair down. So a good night was had by all.

Old Ways, New Ways

We were flying from Alice Springs up to the Barkley Tablelands one time, travelling up there to do some routine medical clinics. I was the pilot and, back in those days, they didn't have telephones out on any of these station properties. Their only communication was by radio. Anyway, the people from this particular cattle station called in to the Alice Springs Flying Doctor Service Base and said that they had an Aboriginal stockman out there who had a severe toothache. So we were flying along and of course we always listened to these sessions because at times you get diversions and so forth.

Anyway, as luck would have it, we were due to be flying over this particular property within about fifteen minutes and we always carried dental gear on the plane with us, just in case. So the doctor got on our radio and said, 'Look, we're on our way up to the Barkley Tablelands but if you bring him out to the airstrip, we'll drop in there in a few minutes, pull the tooth out real quick, then we'll be on our way again.'

So the station people did that. They came out with the biggest, toughest Aboriginal stockman you would ever see and we just opened the back door of the aeroplane and sat him on the floor of the plane, with his feet hanging outside. That was just about the right height for the doctor to get a good grip on a tooth. Then, after we propped up the stockman, the doctor started to get prepared. He decided not to use a needle because it looked like a pretty straightforward extraction and, anyway, we didn't have the time. As you can imagine, with all this going on, it looked a real sight so I decided to take a photograph of the scene. And I was just taking the photo when it all got a bit too much for the big, tough stockman and he passed out.

'Quick, Neil,' the doctor called out, 'grab his head and I'll pull the tooth out while he's unconscious.'

So I grabbed the stockman's head as firmly as I could and held it while the doctor got stuck into it. The only trouble was that the extraction proved to be more difficult than he'd first thought it might be and so he had to push and pull it this way and that until, finally—'pop'—and the tooth came out. Then just after the doctor had extracted the tooth, the stockman began to revive and when he fully came around he found that his aching tooth had disappeared. So he was happy. We were happy. Everyone was happy. Then we just said 'Goodbye' and we jumped back into the plane and we continued on our way, up to the Barkley Tablelands.

So that's just one little story. But, I must say, I liked the Aborigines. And out in some of those old mission and community places, like Papunya and Yuendumu, I took to the old blokes in particular. In fact, I even tried to learn a little bit of the local language and I used to try and talk to the old blokes while the doctors and nurses were running their clinics and taking a look at the crookies—the sick ones. So I met some very interesting characters. I remember, there was one old Aboriginal bloke at Areyonga, who'd apparently been there with Lasseter, when Lasseter went missing out in the Petermann Ranges area, near the eastern border of central Western Australia. And this old fella told me that it's all just a big myth because Lasseter didn't find any gold. In fact, there was no gold out there at all.

And another old bloke, he took a very keen liking to me, probably because I'd taken an effort to learn the language, and I was talking to him one day and he said, 'Ah, Captain we go for a drive.'

'Oh, righto,' I said.

So we hopped in a vehicle and we went for this drive, and we go out onto the flat plains. They're dead flat and, anyway, away in the distance there's some rocks sticking up about twenty foot or so, out of the plain. So we drive over there to these rocks, and in amongst them there's this big cave and we go into the cave and, believe me, it's just a mass of native art. It was absolutely amazing. Stunning. And he just took me there as a favour because he liked me. He trusted me.

And that same old fella, he made me a set of boots that the kadaitcha men wear. Now, so that the kadaitcha men can't be tracked, these boots, they're made out of human hair and emu feathers and blood and stuff. You know the kadaitcha man, don't you? He's the spirit man, the magic man, the one that points the bone. Anyway, this old fella made me these kadaitcha boots and he told me that they'd ward away the evil spirits. So I took them home, and my wife—at that time—she said, 'I'm not gonna to have those smelly things in the house.' And she burnt them. And I reckon that's probably one of the reasons why she's now my ex-wife, because things were never the same after that and so maybe ... just maybe ... the evil spirits got to her after she burnt the boots.

But talking about the kadaitcha men and their magic: we flew out to Papunya Aboriginal Community one day and they'd had a lot of babies dying there. The story was that the kadaitcha man was around, trying to pick out who was behind all the bad medicine that was causing the babies to die. Then, of course, once the kadaitcha man decides who the culprit is, the bloke wakes up with a spear through him, and everything gets back to normal.

Anyway, I don't know what had caused the first few deaths of the babies but because all the Aborigines were so fearful of this kadaitcha man, none of them were game enough to come out of their wurleys or huts. So, by the time we arrived, with everyone being too scared to come out of their wurleys, all these kids had by then begun to suffer from dehydration and so forth. And, over time, until the kadaitcha man found out who was causing all the bad medicine, I think we brought something like about seventeen of these dehydrated kids back into Alice Springs where they could be cared for.

But the Aborigines there were fairly primitive back in those days, back in the fifties and early sixties. Mostly, they still lived by their old ways of thinking. For their birth control, they'd 'whistle-cock' the men. Whistle-cocking's when they make an insertion in the penis and that was their form of birth control: to 'whistle-cock' them.

Oh, I could go on forever with the experiences I had when I was flying out of Alice Springs. I've even got photos of initiation ceremonies, because one time I got an old black fella and I lent him the camera. I mean, he was a terrible photographer but he took all these photos for me and, you know, there wouldn't be too many photographs like that in existence. And, anyhow, when they do these initiation ceremonies, part of it is to do the circumcision. And in the old days they used to get two fairly sharp stones and they'd rub them together and cut the foreskin off. By doing it that way, when they removed the foreskin it sort of sealed off the blood vessels, which was supposed to stop the bleeding.

The only trouble was that they didn't necessarily keep these circumcision stones very clean. Now, I didn't actually see this myself but my predecessor was there when it happened. The doctor at that time was a pom, a chap by the name of Edgar Emerson. Even in the middle of summer, when it was as hot as hell, old Edgar still wore his tweeds and his coat, with the patches on and stuff, and he always wore a tie.

Anyway, my predecessor told me that there was this Aboriginal stockman up at Alexandria Downs Station and, see, the male Aborigines can't get married until they've been initiated and circumcised. So this Aboriginal stockman was in his mid-to-late-twenties and he comes in to see old Edgar and he had a shocking infection in his penis from where they circumcised him. My predecessor reckoned that it was an awful sight, because this fella's penis had swollen up to about three inches round and it'd gone all purple, with pus running out of it everywhere. Anyway, old Edgar took one look at it and he said, 'Oh, good Lord, he's going to lose it.'

And the Aboriginal fella—the one with the infected penis—said to Edgar, 'Oh, yer should'a seen it when it was real crook, doc.'

As I said, I didn't witness that one, thankfully. That was told to me by my predecessor. But, of course, that was the old ways because later on they started using razor blades for circumcision. And they were pretty smart about it too, because what they'd do was they'd carry out the circumcisions just before the Flying Doctor was about to come around on a routine medical visit. Then, when the doctor arrived, the first thing he'd be met with was a line-up of young Aboriginal blokes, all waiting to have their penis cleaned up.

One in a Trillion

I first started flying for the Flying Doctor Service in Alice Springs in the mid-60s, and it was a tremendous experience. At that time they were bringing the Aborigines out of the desert and into settlements because rockets were being launched out of Woomera and they didn't want to hit some poor unfortunate Aborigine who happened to be wandering about out there. When I say 'they', back then I think the ruling organisation was called the Department of Native Affairs.

Anyhow, in those days they were very big on getting the Aborigines vaccinated against everything because having lived out in the wilderness, so to speak, they had no immunity to white fellers' diseases and so forth. So we'd go out to the various missions and communities and places like that. Sometimes we'd even land at a remote cattle station and jump in a vehicle and drive twenty miles or so out to some little Aboriginal camp or other, where the doctors and sisters would jab and record them, and what have you.

See, other than the mass vaccination of the Aborigines, they were also big on recording all their tribal Aboriginal names and who their father was and who their mother was, and that sort of business. But that got a bit confusing after a while because too many of them seemed to have had too many of the same fathers and mothers and everyone else seemed to be known as Aunty Someone-or-other or Uncle Someone-or-other. And that's just the Aboriginal way of family. But it was a real eye-opener because, you know, you'd see all sorts of things; some of the conditions they lived in were indescribable. And the women had legs that were little bigger than broom handles; then sometimes their arms or legs had been broken and had set awkwardly.

But Papunya was probably one of the main places where the Department of Native Affairs brought the Aborigines into. And I'll get a little off the track here and reminisce on a bit and tell you a little story about chance, one that started at Papunya.

We flew into Papunya one time and there was a pregnant nursing sister who worked out there whose name was Marie. Anyway, while the doctor and the nurse were jabbing the Aborigines and recording their names and so forth, I went and had a cup of tea with this Marie. Then a couple of days after I'd flown the doctor and nurse back to Alice Springs, I said to the doctor, 'Gees, I'm itchy.'

'Let's have a look,' he said.

And he just took one look at me and he said, 'You've got German measles. We'll have to go back to Papunya and give an injection of gamma-globulin to all the pregnant women out there, then hope you haven't caused any problems.'

So we went back out to Papunya and, I don't know if you've ever seen it or not, but the gamma-globulin needle is this great, big, long needle which they jab into the rump. It's like a length of no. 8 fencing wire. Anyway, Marie said to me, 'I'm never having another bloody cup of tea with you ever again.'

Unfortunately, in Marie's case she miscarried. She lost the baby.

Then a few years later I got married and at the wedding I was introduced to the in-laws for the first time and my newly acquired sister-in-law looked vaguely familiar. So I said, 'Haven't I seen you before?'

'Yeah,' she said, 'I know you from somewhere, too.'

I said, 'What's your name?'

'Marie,' she said.

And it turned out that this Marie was the same Marie who was the nursing sister out at Papunya, and I was the bloke who caused her to lose her baby because I had German measles. And I'd just married her husband's sister, which made me her brother-in-law. So what's the chances of that happening? About one in a trillion, I'd say.

Pilatus PC 12

I don't think that by me being a female pilot, it changes the way the plane is being flown. In my case it is more working for the Royal Flying Doctor Service that makes an interesting difference to the way I sometimes fly. For an example, it must've been about four or five months ago we were sent to Cook, out on the Nullarbor Plain, for a patient that got sick on the Indian Pacific train. It was a high priority and when we landed the doctor came along and he said, 'Oh, you will have to taxi into town because the patient is too sick to be transported out to the airport.'

Well, the airport was probably about 500 metres or 600 metres from the town but here you go: safety first. Off the airport I went, onto the track and taxi into town and I park the plane under a shady tree. And that's just one of those things you would never come across anywhere else. It was sort of like a special pick-up and it was because, as I said, it was of a very high priority.

It's the same in Tarcoola, which is also out on the Transcontinental Railway Line. When we go there for medical clinics with the GPs, the first time I came there I asked, 'Where do we go?'

And they said, 'Well, you follow the track and you park the aeroplane behind the hospital.'

So those kinds of experiences, of course, are very different to anywhere else with flying, and also much more so because these are usually all-dirt runways.

Another thing that is different is that we all work as a team in the Flying Doctor Service. We all try to help each other. Like what we had in the bush once at William Creek, in the north of South Australia. There was a car rollover after they'd had a heavy night of partying, I think, and we got called out in the very early hours of the morning. But when we got there, to William Creek, we couldn't get the lights to go on, on the airstrip.

But some of the station crew were already out there, because they knew of the emergency and they switched on, manually, the lights of the strip. So you land the aeroplane on the dirt strip and then you help put a stretcher in the back of the good old 'Aussie' ute, jump in the ute, with the nurse and the doctor, drive to where the person is injured and be of any help you possibly can while they get him stabilised and they assess him and things like that. Then you help get him on the stretcher and put the stretcher again in the back of the ute and you drive back to the strip where we then put him on the aircraft and then you take off. So, you know, those are the real stories of accidents in the bush that you can have happen.

One of the first experiences that I had of a night-time flight was with the flares. For those, the RFDS send out forms to all the different stations to show them how to set the flares out and what the procedure is. They give enough light out, but not a whole lot. And with flares, you don't see them until you are only a few miles out from them. So anyway, this time we had to go to Clifton Hills, which is a station property up on the Birdsville Track. It was a pitch black night. There was no moon out, nothing. I was at about 20,000 feet or something and half an hour out from our destination I could look anywhere and I could just not see a single light outside, anywhere. That's how black it was. And I thought, Oh well, this is definitely descending into a black hole.

Anyhow, they set up the flares and then they have a car with the lights that point to where the wind comes from so that you're flying into the wind when you land. So, yeah, that was quite an experience to do that the first time.

But especially when it is totally moonless and you don't have a horizon or anything to look at, because it's just pitch black, then you've really got to be on the ball to do that, because you are virtually just flying by the instruments. Because sometimes you do often hear of that 'black hole' thing—that is when some people can easily lose their direction and also they lose how high they are off the ground, and even whether they're flying up-side-down or not. So you've got to trust your instruments, because in a situation like that what the instruments say can be the opposite to what are our own perceptions. For instance, if you accelerate then your body sensation will say, 'Oh, you're accelerating, so you must be going down.'

That is the feeling you get. Your ears will tell you something different than what your instruments do. It is hard but it's something that you just have to learn—to trust your instruments. So, yeah, black holes can be very dangerous.

But we are very lucky with the Pilatus PC 12 aeroplanes. They've got, for instance, the EGPWS. That stands for Enhanced Ground Proximity Warning System, so that if you're going in on a too-steep approach it will give you little things to warn you that you are too steep. Or when the ground comes up towards you, or you don't have your gear down and your flaps out, and there is a runway, it will go off and say, 'Pull up. Pull up. Terrain. Terrain.'

We also have a multi-function display unit which, at night time, we can use to read the ground, so that we can see where any high areas are. You can sort of see outside, but you can't, if you understand what I mean. But all that works on the display unit, with radar and satellite. So all that instrumentation is of an enormous value to us, especially since we are a single pilot operation.

So the Pilatus PC 12 is a most wonderful aeroplane. In fact, the Flying Doctor Service was one of the first major organisations to use the PC 12s. It is a Swiss-built plane that has got a military background. So they're very well built. But also, I believe the PC 12 was a radical move away from normal thinking because while the King Airs have a twin turbo prop (propeller), the PC 12s have a single engine turbo prop. Of course, with having a single engine, they're a cheaper plane to operate and also they have a shorter landing and take-off length than our King Airs did.

But they are very, very expensive to buy and fit out. I think that I've heard a quote of about six million dollars for each aeroplane. That is with all the medical equipment in them, of course. But they've been a great success, and they suit, very much, our type of work. And I think that now the RFDS, especially in the South Australian or Central Section, has got the highest flight time of PC 12s anywhere in the world.

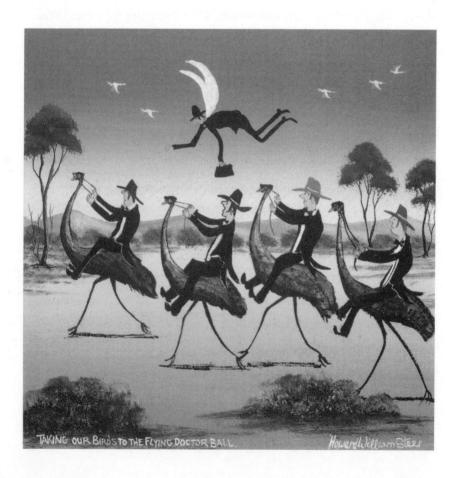

TAKING OUR BIRDS TO THE FLYING DOCTOR BALL.

Preordained Destiny

I was reading your last book of Flying Doctor stories—*More Great Australian Flying Doctor Stories*—and I was particularly taken with a story in there called 'In the Footsteps of Flynn'. In part it describes how Fred McKay's destiny was set out very early on in his life. If you recall, that happened when he was a little boy and he was very ill and he remembered looking up from his sick bed and seeing his mother saying, in silent prayer, 'Lord, if you make my little boy well, I'll make him a minister.'

Of course, we all know now that that's what happened. Fred became a minister and, then, following John Flynn's death, he took over as Superintendent of the Australian Inland Mission. So Fred's destiny was set from a very early age.

Now, I'm not sure if you know but Fred's wife, Meg, also had a very interesting occurrence of preordained destiny. As you know, Meg became such an integral part of Fred's life, not only as his wife but also with the work they both did within the organisation of the AIM. And, well, as it's turned out, I've discovered that that strong connection had its beginnings long before Fred even came along. But putting it all together from my memory is a little hard and of course there's been so much written about both Fred and Meg that it's probably best if you just read about it in a book. It'd be more accurate that way. I mean, as in this case, that's where I came across this particular story about Meg and her destiny. I found it in a very interesting book that was written by Maisie McKenzie. It's called *Outback Achiever: Fred McKay—Successor to Flynn of the Inland*. And this is where a lot of this information comes from, so my apologies to Maisie, but I just want to get it right.

Now, just a bit of background first. Meg was a Robertson, and her father, Hubert Robertson, had been a Presbyterian minister in Scotland. He and his wife were then invited by the Presbyterian Church to come out to Australia; Hubert as an evangelist. That was in 1913. So they settled in Australia and their first daughter, Betty, ended up attending university at the same time Fred was there. I'm not sure just how good friends they were but they knew each other well enough that Fred got to know the Robertson family through his contact with Betty.

Meg was the second daughter. Her given name was Margaret Mary McLeod Robertson or, as she became more commonly known, Meg. Then, later on, when she was at a Presbyterian-Methodist College for girls, that's when she got to know Fred, through his connection with Betty. Now apparently Meg was quite struck by Fred, even back then. But she wasn't sure about Fred's feelings towards her so it came as a real surprise when Fred asked her to accompany him to an Inter-College Boat Race on the Brisbane River. I believe Fred was at Queensland University at Emmanuel College at that stage, studying arts and theology. Now Meg was about eight years younger than Fred so she would've only been, I don't know, about sixteen or seventeen or something. She was still a schoolgirl anyway, and apparently she went off to this boating regatta, along with Fred, all dressed out in the Emmanuel College colours. So she must've been determined to make some sort of an impression.

And that's when they first began to really get to know each other. But at that stage in time they were both so busy, what with Fred and his studies and then, after Meg had finished school, she went to Brisbane to begin her nursing training at the Brisbane Hospital. But her father, Hubert Robertson, had long held a fascination with the work that John Flynn was doing within the AIM, to such an extent that he had then become Chairman of the Queensland Council of the Australian Inland Mission.

Anyway, as the story goes, at one point he had to submit a report to the State Assembly in Brisbane. Meg also attended that State Assembly, along with her family, and she just happened to sit in front of Fred and a group of his college mates. Now, in Maisie McKenzie's book, it says how Fred must've apparently spent more time looking at Meg than he did listening to the Church Fathers, because somewhere during the proceedings he tapped Meg on the shoulder and asked, 'Who's taking you home tonight?'

And, as quick as a flash, Meg replied, 'You are.'

That's when they really first formed their bond because, according to Maisie McKenzie, Fred kissed Meg when they parted that night and I quote 'that marked the beginning of a life-long commitment to each other—one that was to last through the years and lead them on unexpected paths'.

From then on they sort of developed their relationship over the years. I mean, they went to the boat regatta when Meg was about seventeen and they married when she was twenty-two or something like that so they had a reasonably long courtship. That's if you could call it a courtship because they were apart so often. But apparently the kiss sealed it, and from then on they were committed to each other.

Later on, after Fred had graduated, he was appointed to a Home Mission at Southport, on the Gold Coast. The Gold Coast's about a hundred kilometres south of Brisbane. The place suited him well because he liked swimming in the sea and he liked the people. So he was pretty excited about his appointment and he thought he'd settle in there, at Southport, for the next few years. After that his plan was to go overseas to Edinburgh, Scotland, where he wanted to continue with his theological studies.

But while Fred was at Southport, that's when John Flynn came along and asked him to consider becoming a patrol padre, with the AIM. As you've said in your book, Flynn had long been eyeing off Fred as a likely candidate to take over the running of the AIM, after his departure. That part of the story is quite well written about in the story 'In the Footsteps of Flynn', from your book of *More Great Australian Flying Doctor Stories*. You know, with Flynn running some sand through his fingers and saying to Fred, 'The sands of Birdsville are far finer than the sands of Southport' then with Fred following Flynn off the beach and walking in his footsteps as they went.

So that was Fred and his destiny. And now, as I said right at the beginning, there's perhaps an even more interesting story of destiny, hidden in there, within the overall story, and it's about Meg and her long-time connection to the Australian Inland Mission; one that happened long before she met Fred. Now I'd like to quote directly from Maisie McKenzie's book, if I may, because it relates that story far better than what I can tell it.

Okay, so this happened soon after John Flynn had his meeting with Fred on the beach at Southport, with the proposal of him joining the AIM and becoming a patrol padre, out in western Queensland. And I now quote:

And was it in the best interests of the Church and of himself to sacrifice the Edinburgh goal? And what about Margaret Robertson? How would she react? They knew their future was bound together, but Margaret was little more than half-way through her nursing training. He simply had to see her.

He met her at the hospital and they walked in the park, while he told her of the extraordinary experience with John Flynn, who had asked him to be a boundary rider for the Australian Inland Mission and to travel throughout western Queensland. He half expected her to protest that perhaps he was being carried away, or some such thing, but, to his utter astonishment, Margaret unfolded a remarkable story.

She told him that, when her father, Hubert Robertson, had first come out from Scotland as an evangelist, in 1913, the Australian Inland Mission was in its infancy, having started only the year before. But Hubert and his wife read about it and this fascinating, adventurous work in outback Australia captured their imaginations. They found out all they could and, just before Margaret was born in May 1915, they agreed to dedicate the baby, whatever the sex, to the splendid work being carried out by John Flynn and his Australian Inland Mission.

So, even before she was born, Fred's future wife was invisibly bound to the Australian Inland Mission. Six months after her birth, John Flynn, himself, was staying in their [the Robertsons'] Manse. In his usual style he talked late into the night with the eagerly listening Hubert Robertson, telling of his dreams for the future. In the morning he was holding baby Margaret on his lap. Mr Robertson came up to them and placed a one pound note in the baby's hand. 'Now you are a member of the AIM Inland Legion,' he said.

This [the Inland Legion] was an army of voluntary workers in the capital cities, parcelling up literature for the print-hungry people of the inland. A one pound donation gave membership to the Legion. Years after, when Margaret was a grown woman, Flynn told her he had the utmost difficulty in prising that pound note from her tightly clenched fist. She wanted to keep it.

As she [Meg] spoke, Fred could hardly believe his ears. What an amazing coincidence. Or was it? Margaret's story and her enthusiasm clinched it for him, and that was when he made up his mind that he would offer to be Flynn's boundary rider up there in the North, if the AIM wanted him. He says now that he felt as if "the very Spirit of the Lord was speaking, but that this was no still small voice. Rather it sounded like a hammering in my heart".

"But that would mean coming to Birdsville with me when you finish your training," he said.

Margaret, his Meg, a woman in love, replied, "Yes, Birdsville or Edinburgh or Timbuctoo."

I mean, isn't that amazing? And so later on they were married in December 1938. By then Fred was already 'boundary riding' for John Flynn as one of his patrol padres. Then, after they married, Meg started going out on patrol with Fred. Basically, their house was a truck, and they camped out together and stayed at various remote station properties throughout the west of Queensland. And not only did Meg's nursing training come in very handy in that sort of work but she was also given the extra jobs of having to pull teeth out and so forth. Actually, I think she might've even done some sort of a crash course in dentistry because all her old dental instruments have been given to the Fred McKay Museum, there in Alice Springs. So Meg travelled with Fred until their first child, Margaret, was born and so that would've been for another year or year and a half.

But, really, isn't that an amazing coincidence of divine connection? Not only for Fred but for Meg as well, and for both of them to end up becoming life-long partners. I mean, something like that really makes you think about the mysterious ways of preordained destiny, doesn't it?

Razor Blades and Saucepans

Yes now, some of my memories. Well, my flying background goes back to the services. I did my training with the Royal Australia Air Force [RAAF]. That was in 1956, and I served with them for fourteen years. Then, when I got out of the RAAF, I came up to Cairns, in far north Queensland, and joined the Aerial Ambulance crowd. Back then the Aerial Ambulance was operated by the Queensland Ambulance Transport Brigade [QATB], which used to run all the ambulance services throughout the state.

So then I flew with the QATB for about ten years, right up until the middle of 1979, which was when the QATB finally decided to get out of the aeroplane side of things. So I was without a job. Anyhow, out of fifty or so other applicants from all around Australia, I was lucky enough to be picked up by the Royal Flying Doctor Service and based here in Cairns. So I was able to stay here, which was a great relief because when I was in the Air Force, typical military, I'd moved twelve times in fourteen years. Actually, my feeling was that if I never moved again it'd be far too soon. But thankfully as it turned out, I didn't have to move anywhere and I started with the RFDS here in Cairns on the 1st of July, 1979.

And I was with the RFDS then from the middle of 1979 right up until I retired in the middle of 1997 and I was basically based in Cairns for the whole of that time. I was their chief pilot and also their senior checking and training pilot, so that job took me around the ridges a lot, within the confines of the RFDS. You know, I'd find myself out at Charleville and then out at Mt Isa and then down in Brisbane for conferences and all that sort of thing.

Actually, probably the correct sequence should be training and checking pilot, really, but for years and years it's been simpler to just say check and training. And there's a funny little story about that. Years and years ago a crowd called Bush Pilots were operating here in Cairns and they had a fellow who was writing stories about them and he couldn't understand what all this 'check and training' was all about. He thought they were saying 'chicken training'.

'What the hell are you pilots training the chickens to do?' he asked, and it had to be explained that it was actually a process of checking and training pilots, which had nothing at all to do with chicken training.

In those earlier days, of course, there were only the three active bases in Queensland—Cairns, Mt Isa and Charleville—and our Head Office was in Queen Street, Brisbane. Of course, it's all changed now. We still have Cairns, Mt Isa and Charleville but now you've also got Townsville, Rockhampton and Bundaberg and the Head Office has moved from its old place in Queen Street out to the Brisbane Airport. So there's been tremendous changes since I retired.

And, with the clinic flying, which was where we took a doctor and a nurse out to virtually provide a GP service, back then the area we covered was inland from Collinsville, which is between Townsville and Mackay, right up to the top of Cape York. In my day we started on a Tuesday and we'd go from Cairns to Kowanyama, which used to be called Mitchell River. Then from Kowanyama we'd go to Pormpuraaw, which was then known as Edward River. Both Kowanyama and Pormpuraaw are Aboriginal communities. After that we'd go up to Weipa, where we'd overnight, and the next day we'd go down to Aurukun, which is just forty miles south of Weipa. Then we'd fly across to Lockhart River. After Lockhart River we'd go back to Weipa again, to overnight there. Then the following day we might go down to, say, some places like Coen and Musgrave, and then back to Cairns. So it'd be a three-day deal with two nights away from Cairns.

And the aeroplanes we had were the piston-engined Beechcraft Queen Airs. They had those of course before I joined the RFDS in '79. Then, over the years, we progressively phased out the Queen Airs into the turbo prop, Beechcraft King Airs. Gorgeous aeroplanes they were. Simply gorgeous. I really enjoyed flying the King Airs. We got our first one, a King Air Super 200, in 1984, then we subsequently got one, two, three, then four King Air C90s. The C90s were a smaller King Air, based on the Queen Air airframe and they had what was called a 'pumped-up fuselage' [pressurised] and, rather than the piston engines, a couple of turbo prop engines came on it.

Actually, one of the air traffic controllers out in Mt Isa—a lady interestingly enough—described them beautifully, I thought. She'd been watching the Queen Airs take off and land for a number of years and when the first of the little turbo prop King Airs turned up in Mt Isa she said it was like a 'Queen Air with balls'. And I still haven't heard it put any better than that.

So then there was sort of a phasing-out period of the Queen Airs, where we went from having four Queen Airs to having three Queen Airs to having two Queen Airs to having one. Actually, I flew the last Queen Air. From memory, I think that was in May 1992 and it finished up as an exhibit in our RFDS visitor's centre, here in Cairns.

So the last of our Queen Airs still exists, thank goodness. They were going to chuck it out but I prevailed upon them. I made the very strong suggestion that we really should try and retain some of our own aviation history. To my way of thinking, Australia was far too keen on discarding its older aeroplanes to turn them all into razor blades and saucepans. And of course nowadays everyone's running around trying to find old World War II aeroplanes, you know. And, mind you, that's only just sixty years after the event. But that's another story.

See Yer Later

Now, I've only got just the one Flying Doctor story, so I don't know if it's of use to you.

Okay, well some years ago, after exploring Ningaloo Reef, between Exmouth and Coral Bay, which is up in the northern coastal region of Western Australia, we headed off to Exmouth Airport, with our dive bags and packs, to catch a small plane to Broome. When we arrived at Exmouth, there were only a couple of four-wheel drives in the airport car park. Then, further to that, we discovered that the actual terminal was completely deserted; that is, except for one bloke who was behind a check-in counter.

'G'day,' we said.

'Oh, glad you've turned up,' he beamed. 'You're the only passengers for the day!'

'What? No one else here?' I asked.

'No,' he replied, 'just the bloke in the Control Tower.' Then he gave us the tags to stick on our luggage. 'Here,' he said, 'stick these on your bags and have a good flight.'

Which we did and then, to our surprise, he slipped under the counter and headed out to the car park. So we settled into these terribly bright red seats that were in the waiting lounge. To give you some idea, they were a kind of a cross between a beanbag and a park bench-seat. In actual fact, the whole terminal was done out in probably what some people would call 'post-modern'. But at least the windows were huge, even if the runway and tarmac were totally deserted.

So, anyway, we sat and we waited. And we sat and we waited, and the departure time for our six-seater came and went. Then eventually we heard a plane. As the plane landed and taxied to the terminal, we read 'Royal Flying Doctor Service' on the side of it. Of course, this obviously wasn't our Broome service. Anyhow, the instant the engines died a young woman dressed in uniform jumped out of the plane and she started running towards the terminal. At seeing her urgency and sensing an emergency, I went over to meet her at the gateway.

'I'm sorry,' I said, 'but we're the only people here, except for the bloke in the Control Tower.'

'No worries,' she said, 'I'm just busting for a piss.' And she keep on running, straight towards the toilet.

So I went and sat back down again. Then she emerged a little later, looking far more relaxed, and she walked sedately over to us.

'So where are you going?' she asked.

'Broome,' we said.

'Bad luck,' she said, 'we're heading the other way.'

'Oh,' we said.

Then she said, 'See yer later then,' and rushed back out to the RFDS plane, jumped back in, and they took off.

Speared

Well, I joined the Flying Doctor Service in 1989. That was as a pilot out at Meekatharra, which is in the central-west of Western Australia. Then, after about six months at Meekatharra, in early May 1990 I went to work up at their Port Hedland Base. I stayed at Port Hedland then for thirteen years, until 2003, and oh, we loved it there. We had a young family and it was such a good, safe place to bring up kids. We also loved camping so there was lots of bush trips and travelling around the Pilbara and the Kimberley. The Gibb River Road's one of my favourite places in Australia. Actually, I think we've done the Gibb River Road about six times and I reckon there's still more to see. Fabulous country up that way. In fact, just about my whole flying career has taken place throughout the tropical areas of Australia. You know, northern Western Australia right across to northern Queensland.

But as far as stories go, you always sort of have your favourites, don't you? One that I think was quite amusing in an odd sort of way—well, both sad and amusing, I guess— happened at Jigalong Aboriginal Community. Jigalong's about 120 kilometres east of the mining town of Newman, in central Western Australia.

Anyhow, once every two or three years the Aborigines conduct what's called Law Ceremonies. Now, these Law Ceremonies happen when all the various communities from within the wider area gather together in a designated community and, along with a lot of celebrations, the Elders review events since the last get-together. So they'd do things like the initiations with the young boys who haven't yet been initiated, and also they'd deal out the tribal punishment for any misdemeanours or whatever that may have occurred over the last couple of years or so. So you could do something wrong and then you might have to wait for a year or more before you got punished, in the appropriate law time.

On this particular occasion there'd been a car rollover and two passengers had been killed and so the driver of the vehicle was brought before the Elders. The Elders listened to what had happened and deemed that it was the driver's fault for causing the deaths of the two others. So he had to be punished and the Elders said that his punishment was to be a stabbing in the thigh, by a spear.

So a few men grabbed hold of the bloke who'd been driving the car and they held him as still as they could, ready to receive the punishment. But apparently the driver bloke was wriggling and turning and writhing around so much that the enforcer of the punishment clean missed his mark and he ended up spearing the driver bloke in the lower abdomen instead of the thigh.

That's when we got an emergency call to go out there to Jigalong Community to pick up the bloke who'd been speared. The only trouble was that, unfortunately, it'd been raining heavily over the area for the past week or so and there was no way we could land the aeroplane on Jigalong airstrip.

But, seeing that it was an emergency, they arranged to charter a helicopter from Karratha. The helicopter was then flown up to Newman and we took the RFDS aeroplane down from Port Hedland, where we all got into the helicopter and we flew out from Newman to Jigalong. Along with the helicopter pilot we took the normal complement of RFDS staff, which was a doctor, the nurse and myself.

And so we went out in the chartered helicopter and landed at the local oval, at Jigalong Community, and they brought out the poor guy who'd been inadvertently speared in the lower abdomen. We quickly laid him on the stretcher, put him onto the helicopter and took him back to Newman. The helicopter then headed back to Karratha and we put the speared bloke into the RFDS aeroplane and flew him back to Port Hedland, where he was going to be treated.

Then we'd only just arrived back in Port Hedland when we got another call asking us to return to Jigalong Community. Apparently, what happened was that the Elders had gone and handed out another punishment and that person had been speared, this time in the thigh. Anyhow, I think that in the end they decided that his new bloke's wounds weren't quite bad enough to warrant us going through the whole procedure again. You know—of chartering another helicopter to fly out there and for us to fly down to Newman, and all that. I mean, the cost was astronomical. I'd estimate that just that one retrieval cost would've been well over $30,000.

But the irony of the whole thing was that we later found out that the second call for us to return to Jigalong Community was to pick up the bloke who'd inadvertently stuffed up the first spearing. Apparently the Elders deemed that he should be punished for being such a poor shot.

Stroke

I've got a couple of stories about sort of strokes here, if you like. Well, for a few seasons I worked out at Mulga Downs Station, cooking for the jackeroos and all that. Mulga Downs is just north of Wittenoom, in northern Western Australia. Anyhow, I had a little medical knowledge—not much, but a little—and one time I was out there and the station manager's wife came and woke me up in the middle of the night. 'My husband's having a stroke,' she said.

Well, she thought he was having a stroke, anyway. So I went over to the homestead and the manager was lying on the bed with his legs crossed. To my thinking that didn't really look like he was having a stroke. But he said that he had all these spots in front of his eyes and when he'd tried to get up to go to the toilet he couldn't walk. He was also in terrible pain and was feeling sick in the stomach.

Anyway, I called the Flying Doctor Base in at Port Hedland and the doctor there asked if I could give the manager an injection of stemetil, out of the homestead's RFDS medical chest, and also some pethidine if necessary. Stemetil is what you have for nausea. Pethidine is for the pain. So I gave the manager an injection of stemetil, which seemed to settle him down a bit. I didn't want to give him the pethidine just then, because I knew it'd mask the cause of whatever his pain was and that'd only make the doctor's diagnosis more difficult. So I kept the pethidine with me in my hand, but only to use if necessary, as I thought it'd be better to try and wait until the doctor came and had a good look at him.

Now, because Mulga Downs only had a small airstrip which could only be used during the day, the Flying Doctor suggested that they meet us out at the Auski Roadhouse. The Auski Roadhouse is on the Great Northern Highway between Newman and Port Hedland. They had an airstrip near the roadhouse there, where the Flying Doctor could land at night. So we rang the Auski Roadhouse to let them know what was going on and asked if they could get somebody to go out and light the lamps along the airstrip. We then loaded the crook manager into the vehicle and drove him the forty or so kilometres from Mulga Downs to the Auski Roadhouse.

Anyway, the Flying Doctor arrived at Auski and they took him straight back to Port Hedland. But as it turned out, what the manager had was a severe migraine. So it wasn't a stroke, it was a severe migraine. Then the next day, the manager's wife had to go over to Port Hedland and bring him home, and he was okay after that.

Now, to the next story about a stroke, and this was a real stroke. Again I was working out at Mulga Downs Station. The station manager and his wife were going on holiday and they'd organised for their homestead to be painted while they were away. So they asked if I'd come out a little earlier than usual that season and cook for the house painter plus Arthur, the guy who was looking after the windmills, while they went on holidays. That was fine by me and I headed out to Mulga Downs.

For the life of me I can't recall his name just now, but anyhow, there was the painter, Arthur and myself. That's all. It was stinking hot and the three of us were staying in the one cottage because it was the one that had cooling. Then early one morning, around four o'clock, I got woken up by the painter feller banging on my wall. 'Get Arthur,' he was calling out. 'Get Arthur, I've had a stroke.'

Luckily, he could still talk. So I went in to check on him and there he was, lying on the floor, paralysed down one side. I then went and woke Arthur up and he came in and looked after the painter while I went over to the homestead and called the Flying Doctor. They said that it'd take two hours for them to fly from Port Hedland, out to the small airstrip at Mulga Downs, and pick up this painter feller.

With that done I went back to the cottage to see how the painter was getting on and, oh, he was really worried because he said that he had all his money stashed away in his car. You know how pensioners save up their money; like they put it under the mattress and in odd places like that. Well, this bloke had all his money hidden in his car and he wanted me to go and get it for him, which I did. It was a fair bit of cash too; in the thousands. So it was a lot of money.

When I came back, I gave the money to the painter. 'Thanks,' he said, but, by now, he wasn't looking too well at all; his condition had deteriorated.

Anyhow, I took over looking after him then, while Arthur went and cleaned out the back of a ute so that we could fit the stretcher in. It was just on daylight by now and we knew that the Flying Doctor wouldn't be too far away. So we loaded the painter in the back of the ute and we went down to the airstrip. The kangaroos were particularly bad just on dawn and so the next thing we had to do was to drive up and down the airstrip in an attempt to scare them off. By that stage the painter was going from bad to worse. He kept stopping breathing on me, and even more worrying was that I could see that his hand was clenching. That's a bad sign. So while Arthur was driving up and down the airstrip, I just had to sit there in the back of the ute, continually wiping the painter's face with a wet cloth in an attempt to at least keep him comfortable.

By the time the Flying Doctor arrived it was daylight, and what a welcoming sight that was, I can tell you. The plane landed and the doctor comes down—mind you, he's just dressed in a shirt and shorts, and he also brings the daily paper, for good measure—and the first thing he said was, 'We've been trying to call you on the radio. Why didn't you answer?'

'Well,' I said, 'I couldn't because someone had to stay with the patient.'

Anyway, when the Flying Doctor took the painter's blood pressure it was up around, something like, 210 over 100 and, you know, normal is somewhere down around 120 or 130. So they quickly loaded him into the plane and flew him back to Port Hedland.

I'm not really sure what happened to the painter after that because I ended up leaving Mulga Downs, though I don't think he ever came back to pick up his car. The station manager later told me that he'd had another stroke and had lost the power of speech. He might've even ended up in Rehab or somewhere. But I've often wondered whatever happened to all that cash of his that I handed over to him, on the night of his first stroke. I'll never know. And so I guess that no one else will ever get to know about it either.

Stuck

One of the worst things that ever happened was when I was driving this very ill lady, Dorethea, in our old ambulance down to Newman, in the central north of Western Australia. Dorethea was one of the great characters of Wittenoom. But then, well, the ambulance broke down, didn't it? Poor old Dorethea, by that stage she'd been projectile vomiting for days and was extremely dehydrated and we only found out later that she had a blocked intestine.

By that stage I'd already called the Flying Doctor Service but they couldn't come out because the RFDS plane was busy, down in Perth. See, there'd been this big accident out on the Newman road where a man and his daughter and, I think, the daughter's friend were all killed. But anyway, someone was also very badly injured in that accident and the RFDS had flown the badly injured person down to Perth. That's why they couldn't get out to us. So, with Dorethea in such a bad state, and with the RFDS plane in Perth, that left us with no other choice than to drive her over to Newman for medical help.

Anyhow, you wouldn't believe it, but about sixteen kilometres out of Wittenoom the wheel bearing went on the ambulance. It was almost midnight by then and because it was such an old ambulance, the radio wouldn't work either. So the girl I had along with me, Julie, she decided to walk on the gravel road, in the dark, back to Wittenoom to get help. And that was one of the scariest things because after Julie left I was stuck out there alone, with Dorethea. And, you know, I'm only a volunteer ambulance officer. I'm not qualified, and here's Dorethea vomiting and going into shock, you know. I was giving her sips of water, which she was bringing straight up. They later told me I shouldn't have given her anything but, you know, in a case like that, you don't know what you're supposed to do, do you really?

I remember that it was a warm night and there was no moon, nothing, just really low cloud. So it was really dark. So we were just stuck there and then the lights went out in the ambulance. The battery went flat because I'd had the lights on. That's probably because it was only ever used once in a blue moon and the battery wasn't strong enough. So there I am; I'm there with only the torch light, trying to read the First Aid Manual to see what to do with someone who's in shock and is projectile vomiting at the same time. Oh my God, it was terrible. I really thought she was going to die. I tell you, we both needed all the help we could get so we both decided to pray, together.

Anyhow, I stayed with Dorethea, just hoping and praying for somebody to come along. But they didn't ... well, not for four hours, anyway. By then Julie had walked back to town and woken somebody up. Then, when we eventually got rescued, we took Dorethea back to town. Someone had called the Flying Doctor again and by that time the plane was on its way back from Perth. So then they came up and we sent her by plane to Port Hedland. So the RFDS had a busy night as well.

Then after going to Port Hedland, Dorethea ended up in Perth and eventually she died. And, you know, I was so worried that I'd done something wrong, especially as I knew her so well. I even ended up calling the Perth Hospital and asking them about it, and they said, 'No, it wasn't from any of your neglect or anything. It was because she had this blocked intestine.'

Mind you, she was also seventy-two by that stage and she'd smoked unfiltered cigarettes all her life and drank wine every day. But it took me a long time to get over that. A very long time. So that was another corker.

Still, I did the best I could and I guess you can't do any more than your best, can you?

That's My Job

I came up to the Kimberley area, in the north of Western Australia, back in 1969 as a lay missionary for the Catholic Church and I worked at St Joseph's Hostel, here in Derby, where we looked after about eighty children. Actually, St Joseph's Hostel burnt down about five or six years or so ago but it used to be up on the corner there. Then I got married to Colin in '73 and we worked out on Mt Barnett Station for the first year of our marriage. After that we went to Gibb River Station, and we stayed there for a total of twenty-six years.

Actually, Colin's family owned Gibb River Station. His father started it in 1922 and we ended up eventually selling it to the Aboriginal people in 1989. Basically, we sold it because, by that time it had four families to support which naturally made it a bit hard to manage. As you might realise, the pastoral industry's not that strong these days and out there it's marginal country, anyway. I mean, it's quite big because it's something like a million acres but you've only got, like, 6000 head of cattle. That's about all it can take.

Anyway, as I said, in 1989 we sold Gibb River Station to the Aboriginal people and they asked Colin and his older brother, Frederik, if they could stay on to help them manage the place. They also wanted help to set up the community in conjunction with the Aboriginal and Torres Strait Islander Commission, or ATSIC as it's known. So we did that, and Frederik stayed on for three years, I think it was, and then we stayed on for a further eight years after Frederick left. So that was about eleven years in all that we remained there, after selling the property. And over the years we were out there we went from a little 5 KVA generator to the bigger ones like the 3 x 70 KVA generator. And I think something like sixteen houses were built in that time, plus the medical clinic, which the RFDS used to service.

Along with all that, the Catholic Church also became involved. I think they were there for ten years or so before we left. Well, they came in with two nuns from New Zealand and they built a beautiful school there and two houses for the nuns. The school always had about twenty kids in it and it was run very well.

Then we left in 2000. We'd been out there for twenty-six years by then, and we were ready to come into town. Well, it was just circumstances really, and it felt like it was time to leave. We'd already bought a property in Derby five years prior to that, but we'd rented it out. It's one of those five acre blocks out on the Gibb River Road. They call them the Gibb River blocks. And it was quite funny really because just the year before we left Gibb River Station, to come into town to live, the base administrator's job here at the Derby RFDS was advertised and the instant I saw it I said to Colin, 'That's my job.'

But, see, we didn't come into town that year. So I was a little bit disappointed about that because I really thought it was a job that I'd like to do and one I was also well suited to do. Of course, by that stage I already had a strong connection with the Flying Doctor Service because when we were out on Gibb River Station, we used them quite a lot. Well, Gibb River had up to 120 people on the property—Aboriginal people, mainly—and I'd helped set up the medical clinic there during our last five or so years. Then we also had the standard RFDS medical chest on the property, which I was responsible for, and we were forever calling them for different things. Oh, well, it was mainly just run-of-the-mill stuff, like accidents, falls off horses, sick kids and all that kind of thing. So, having had to use them so much when we were out on the station, I already had a strong affiliation with the RFDS.

And then, as luck would have it, the next year after we'd moved into town, the same base administrator's job came up. So I applied for the position and got it. And I was really pleased about that because, as I said, when it had originally come up, I felt that it was definitely 'my job'. And now I've worked here at the RFDS in Derby since October 2000. As far as my responsibilities go, we've got fifteen houses for staff, so I look after all the housing. I also combine the three base rosters from the doctors, pilots and nurses and do all the invoicing. I also enter the remote 'consults' [consultations] on the computer data for funding purposes and records. And that's about it really, other than, of course, lots of other little bits and pieces of jobs thrown in. So, basically, what I tell everyone is that, 'I mainly try to keep 'em all happy. That's my job.'

The Normanton Bell

I guess that you've heard about how it was John Flynn who first set up the Australian Inland Mission [AIM] and then the Royal Flying Doctor Service came out of that. But, anyway, the AIM not only sent out nurses and that to remote parts of Australia, there was also a more spiritual side to it and so John Flynn used to send out padres to various parts of the land and it was their job to 'keep an eye on His flock', so to speak.

So that's a bit of the background to this story and, as I've already told you in my book *Goldie*, I was working up in the Gulf one time, doing a bit of this, that and the other, plus doing a bit of cattle duffing on the side. Right, so I'm back in Normanton, staying out with the Caseys. The Caseys were big cattle duffers up that way. So I was staying with them. They owned a place called Shady Lagoons. Anyhow, I'd come into town from Shady Lagoons and I was drinking with a feller by the name of Jack McNab. Jack was a saddler and he also had a mail run. So me and him, we're up in the top pub—the National Hotel—and we'd been drinking on and off all the afternoon. You know, we weren't downing them one after the other like, we were just drinking nice and steady. Anyhow, by about ten o'clock that night, Jack and me, we're starting to get a bit argumentative with each other and this argument's getting pretty warmed up. I forget what it was about just now, but it was heating up.

Anyhow, Sam Henry, the local sergeant, comes in. Sam's the feller who refereed that fight with me and Ronny Paul. Yeah, so Sam Henry comes in and he's sitting down the other end of the bar and he's thinking, Gees, it looks like a blue's on the cards here between Goldie 'n McNab. So Sam comes up and he goes through all the change we had on the counter and he hands it over to Ted Kershaw, the publican. 'Ted,' he says, 'give us a dozen beers.' In those days all the beer was in 26 ounce bottles. The big ones. There was no stubbies.

So Ted goes and he gets the beer, see. 'Here yer go,' he says, and he hands it over to Sam Henry.

Then Sam says to me and Jack, 'Righto, youse fellers, come with me,' and he puts the carton on his shoulder and he walks out of the pub. So me and Jack, we follow him out. By now, me and Jack, we're just talking and going on. There's no arguing, we're just talking.

So then Sam gets in his vehicle. It's a ute sort of thing and Jack and me, we get in the back and Sam drives us out to the edge of town to an old timber church. Now, this old church was built round the turn of the century, back in the early 1900s. It'd weathered a lot of cyclones so it's leaning over at about a thirty degree angle. It was one of them old weatherboard ones that's up on stumps; you know, with the white ant caps on top. They didn't even hold services there any more because there wasn't much floorboards left. Like, anybody in town who wanted a bit of timber always went down to the old church to get it. Yeah, that's where they went for their timber.

So Sam drops me and Jack off out there, at this old church, with this dozen beers. Now, outside the front of the church, about thirty feet or something, there was still the original old bell and this old bell had a length of rope hanging off it.

Any rate Sam plonks us there and he says, 'Righto, fellers, go fer yer life. Do what yer like', then he jumps back in his car and he goes back to town.

So me and Jack, we're left sitting there. We'd both long forgot what the argument was about, so now we're bored and we're looking for something to do. And, see, around Normanton there's a lot of goats walking around all the time. So I says to Jack, I says, 'Let's have some fun. We'll catch a goat 'n tie his back leg ter the rope on the bell, 'n as he's trying ter get away he'll be ringin' the bell.'

'Okay,' Jack says, and so we tried to catch one of these goats, ay, but we're too drunk to catch a goat. They kept getting away from us.

'This's no good,' I says to Jack. 'We're gettin' nowhere. So how's about we ring the bell ourselves?'

'Yeah,' he says. 'Good idea.'

So I start ringing this bell, ay. By now it's about two o'clock in the morning, and we're ringing away and we can see all these house lights being turned on around town, left, right and centre. Now at that time there was only one minister in Normanton. I forget his name just now, but he was what they called a 'padre' because he belonged to the Australian Inland Mission. Anyhow, he lived a way over on the other side of Normanton. A way over. So I must've been making a real racket, ay, because next thing this padre comes flying down in his car.

I says, 'Oh, how yer goin', Padre? Have a drink.'

But he's in no mood for that, ay, because he gives us this big lecture on the evils of drinking. Then he says, 'You shouldn't be ringin' that bell.'

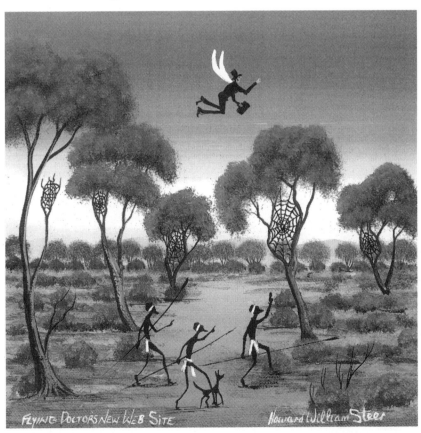

FLYING DOCTORS New WEB SITE   Howard William Steer

I says, 'Why's that?'

He says, 'Because when a church bell's rung, it's meant to be the call for all sinners to come to church.'

So I says, 'Well, this must be a pretty righteous town, ay, Padre?'

'Why's that?'

I says, 'Because you're the only person who's turned up.'

After that he sort of gave up on us and he got back in his car and he drove back into town. So that's the story of the Normanton bell and the AIM padre.

The 'Singing'

I'll never forget the first trip I did, from Alice Springs out to Yuendumu Aboriginal Community, as a pilot with the Flying Doctor Service. I remember we pulled up at Yuendumu and the doctor took one look out the plane window and he said, 'Jesus, there's something strange going on here.'

And he was right, too. You wouldn't believe it: all the Aboriginal men were over in one group and all the women and the kids were in another group and they were all wailing. Gees, it was a real eerie, haunting sort of sound, you know, like, 'Woo … woo … woma, woma … woo.' And when you've got a whole mob of people wailing like that, it makes a fair bit of noise.

Anyway, they had two nursing sisters working there and one of the sisters came over and she explained that the Aborigines were 'singing' a young bloke, for pinching the Tjuringa Stones. You know what the Tjuringa Stones are, don't you? They're the sacred stones. They're like how we keep a history book or a diary; well, they actually etch their stories into these stones. If you ever see them, they've got circles and all sorts of patterns etched on them. It could be all about some big meeting or a corroboree or some sort of gathering or anything. And they treasure these Tjuringa Stones and they bury them in a special place, somewhere safe like a cave or somewhere like that.

I've got one, actually. An old Aboriginal fella gave me one and I never worked out why he gave it to me, because he wasn't really a bloke I knew that well. But, with me being a pilot with the Flying Doctor Service, he knew who I was, of course, and one day he just came up and he gave me this string of stones. If I showed it to you I wouldn't be able to tell you what the story's about. But they know. And my wife won't touch them. They scare her. She reckons I should give the thing back to them, and she's probably right.

But anyhow, so this young Aboriginal fella at Yuendumu, Leo his name was. They used to call him 'Useless Leo'. Leo was only about seventeen and what he'd done was, he'd pinched these Tjuringa Stones and he was going to sell them on the open market. See, being a one-off, they'd be worth quite a few bob; perhaps a couple of hundred thousand dollars or maybe more if he sold them to someplace like a museum. Of course, he'd have to have contacts to sell them to a place like that. So someone might've even put him up to it. I don't know.

Anyway, they caught Leo pinching these Tjuringa Stones and so they 'sung' him, which was like putting a death curse on him. It's similar to pointing the bone.

So the doctor said, 'Okay, after we've finished our routine medical visit here, we'd better get this Leo on the plane and take him back to Alice Springs.'

Now, the doctor had a plan. See, it's all psychological, and that plan was to collect some old stones and a bit of wire and things like that, and when he got Leo in the plane he'd put him under anaesthetic to knock him out. Then, while Leo was out to it, the doctor was going to make a superficial cut across his stomach and when Leo woke up he'd simply hand Leo the wire and stones and stuff and say, 'There you go, Leo. I've just operated on you and I've got all the "bad stuff" out, so now you'll be okay.'

That sort of thing had worked before on a few occasions and when the Aboriginal fellas take a look at the wire and stones, they think, Oh, I'm cured now. The doctor's got all the bad stuff out that the witch doctor had done to me. And then they're fine.

So that's what the doctor was going to do this day. And when Leo walked onto the aircraft he was as fit as a fiddle. He was scared, naturally, but he was medically okay. It was only an hour-and-a-half flight back to Alice Springs and he'd died by the time we were landing in Alice Springs. The doctor told me that he'd been trying to get an adrenalin shot into Leo's veins, but he said it was like trying to put a needle into a piece of string because all Leo's veins had collapsed from the shock of him being 'sung'.

Now, I don't know if you believe in those sorts of things— like pointing the bone and being 'sung'—but Leo certainly must've believed in it. Amazing, isn't it? He walked on the aircraft, unaided, and he was dead within an hour and a half.

The Sweetest Sound

I would like to tell you just the one story. It may be a little bit long-winded but it's a magnificent story I believe, because it was something that personally happened to me. When I first joined the Royal Flying Doctor Service, about ten years ago, I went out on a clinic run and we flew out to a property called the Pinnacles, which is up in the Cape York area of Queensland.

Now, if I could just sort of set the scene for you. As the aircraft landed at the Pinnacles I looked at the four horizons. It was the dry season so it was a pretty dry and unforgiving land that stretched out before me. In fact, there was a cruelty and harshness about it. But, given all that, I suppose the emotions that went through my mind at that particular time were of an overriding beauty. And I suppose that it was my first realisation or understanding of where the great architects of verse—the likes of Banjo Paterson and Henry Lawson and Dorothea Mackellar and so forth—got their inspiration to write about this wonderful land of ours.

But, even apart from that, I felt rather blessed because after we flew in, the original white pioneers of the Pinnacles were there to visit the Flying Doctor. As I said, it was a clinic trip and these two people had long retired. In fact, they were well into their eighties at this time, and they needed to see the doctor on that day. So they were there, waiting, and it was just a marvellous coincidence that I was there to meet them. And while I was looking out at, you know, these barren never-never lands of ours, I happened to say to the old man, 'Just what gave you the fortitude to come out here?'

And without hesitation he simply replied, 'The Flying Doctor.'

And it was at that moment the penny dropped, because I remember many years ago I either read it or heard the words of a speech that Sir Robert Menzies made when he was Prime Minister. And Sir Robert Menzies said something along the lines of, 'The greatest single contribution to the development of inland Australia was Flynn's Flying Doctor Service.' And it hadn't really sunk in until I was standing there with these two old pioneers at the Pinnacles.

But what was to really blow me away, was a statement that I'll basically take to the grave with me, because it was just so wonderful. This old man's beautiful old wife, she looked at me and she said, 'Stephen, the sweetest sound in all the world is the sound of the Flying Doctor aircraft overhead.'

When she said that I conjured up a mental image of her as a young lady giving birth to their first child. So I verbalised that to her and she gave me a bit of a wise smile and said, 'Yes, you're right, that certainly was a pretty tough time and the Royal Flying Doctor Service got me through that one okay.' Then she went on to say, 'But, really, it was many years later when our eldest son was about thirteen and he'd fallen from his horse.' And she pointed to the ground, only metres from where we were standing, and she said, 'I sat right over there and I cradled my precious son's unconscious head in my lap and I cried and I prayed and I cried and I prayed and then I heard the Flying Doctor aircraft overhead. That was the sweetest sound.'

Well, honestly, let me say that when a beautiful old pioneering lady tells a new chum on the block a story like that, well, she truly reached forward and indelibly touched my soul. And, you know, in various fundraising appeals now, for many years, the RFDS has used her statement, because it pretty much depicts, I think, how a lot of people out in those remote lands feel about the Flying Doctor Service.

The Wrong People

Actually, I was up in Whyalla for ten years, working as a pilot with Air Ambulance, before I was transferred to Adelaide. Then I guess I was probably only down here for twelve months or less when they decided it'd be a much better set-up if Aero-medical and the Royal Flying Doctor Service came under the one umbrella. I think it all might've had something to do with the way both the federal and state funding bodies worked. But it wasn't really such a big difference for us because the pilots with Air Ambulance just changed uniforms and became Flying Doctor pilots. It was as simple as that, and that would've been around 1990. So you could say that I'm in about my sixteenth year with the Flying Doctor Service, as such, but I was with Air Ambulance ten years prior to that. So that's twenty-six years in all, which is a fair time.

But it's really a fascinating job. Of course, like any type of employment it has its ups and downs. Probably its biggest drawback is the rotating shift work. That gets you down occasionally, because with the longer shifts we're actually on page [on call] at home for a twelve-hour period and if it is a Code One or a retrieval we've only got forty-five minutes from the time we get paged to 'doors closed' in the aircraft. That means that, virtually, you've got to be in your uniform at all times because when you get paged you have to drive to the airport, get the forecast, check the aircraft and everything and be ready within that forty-five-minute time frame. Of course, if it's just a normal routine-type transfer, you get more time and that's sixty minutes' notice.

A normal type transfer would be, say, taking a patient from somewhere like Port Augusta Hospital to the Royal Adelaide Hospital, as well as transferring people back home. To some it may sound a little bit odd to be using an expensive aircraft for moving people around like that but in reality it's probably more feasible to do it by air than by road. Because, firstly, it's important for the road ambulances and their crews to remain stationed within their community, just in case there's a disaster or something. And, secondly, if an ambulance crew's driving someone from Port Lincoln to Adelaide, they'd have to travel during the day, overnight in Adelaide, then drive back home the next day. So the community would be without an ambulance, effectively, for two whole days. Whereas if you're using an aircraft, in a normal shift we might fit three of those type of transfers in. So really, by using the aeroplane you're saving up to six days work for an entire ambulance crew. What's more, it's less stressful for the patient to travel by air.

But the patients don't know all that. I mean, sometimes they don't even realise they're going to travel with us. They may think they're going by road but the ambulance only takes them as far as the local airstrip where they're loaded onto the aircraft.

Though you do get some mix-ups. Now, I won't mention any names of course, but some years ago one of our pilots flew over to Kingscote, on Kangaroo Island, in South Australia, to pick up a patient. So he gets to Kingscote and he lands and he's greeted by a despondent looking ambulance crew.

'Where's the patient?' the pilot asks.

'Sorry,' they said, 'we haven't got him.'

'What do you mean, you haven't got him?' the pilot asked.

'He escaped from the hospital and we can't find him.'

So the pilot had to turn around and go back to Adelaide without the patient.

And there's another one that I think was extremely funny— and I must stress that this was back before Aero-medical came under the umbrella of the Royal Flying Doctor Service. I just want to make that nice and clear. Anyhow, the chaps from Air Ambulance were asked to fly down to Hamilton, in south-western Victoria, to pick up two patients and bring them back to Adelaide for some minor treatment or other. These two people were 'sitting patients', which means they weren't serious cases so they could make their own way out to the airstrip, without the need for an ambulance. Anyhow, the instruction came through that these patients would be waiting for the plane to arrive.

Now, I don't know if you've ever been to the Hamilton airstrip or not but back in those days there wasn't much there. Anyhow, they'd just landed the Chieftain at Hamilton when these two people walked across to the aircraft and said, 'Have you come to pick us up?'

There was nobody else about so the pilot and the nurse said, 'Yes. Hop in.'

So they loaded the two patients into the plane, where they were made nice and comfortable. 'Thank you. Thank you,' they kept saying. 'You're very kind.'

Then just after they took off, one of the passengers leaned over to the pilot and said, 'So, what's the weather going to be like in Melbourne today?'

'Melbourne?' asked the pilot.

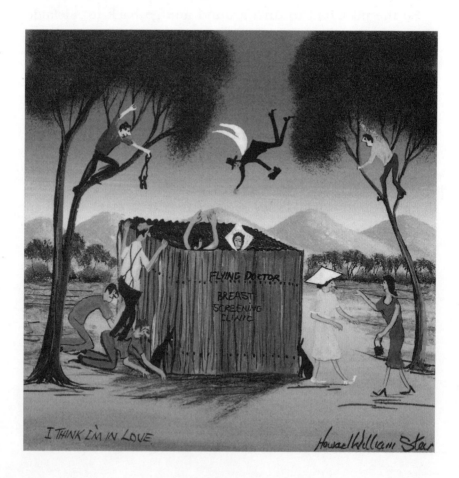

'Yes, we've purchased two tickets to fly over to Melbourne to do some shopping.'

So it was a case of, 'Oops, we've obviously picked up the wrong two people.'

Things that Happened

On 21 August 2001 the Guild of Air Pilots and Air Navigators Association awarded me a Master Air Pilot Certificate—No. 868—which, as it states, is 'awarded in recognition of skill, experience and service in the profession of aviation'. In all, I was a pilot for over forty years, and twenty-one of those were with the Royal Flying Doctor Service. So would you like to hear about some of the things that happened when I was with the RFDS? I've got a few notes already written down here that Bob Rogers, the ex-President of the Royal Flying Doctor Service in Queensland, requested for his book on the organisation. Now, I'm not a great storyteller, as such, so do you mind very much if I pretty much read from what I wrote for Bob's book?

Okay, I suppose there's been many memorable, and not so memorable, incidents that have happened over the twenty-one years I was flying with the Royal Flying Doctor Service. But, as is my way, I've never been one to be totally governed by rules and regulations. That's just not me. So I've been hauled over the coals by the DCA [Department of Civil Aviation] on a few occasions, perhaps the most ironic being one time out at Jundah.

Jundah's in south-western Queensland and we were called out there to pick up a patient who was suffering the

DTs (delirium tremens) due to the severe effects of alcohol consumption. Because of this condition, the patient was quite difficult to handle and by the time we talked the person into getting on the aircraft an approaching dust storm had turned things quite dark. So it was a very big dust storm. Anyhow, I wasn't unduly bothered because, as was normal in such situations, I organised for some cars to light up the airstrip and, along with the aircraft lights, we took off safely and the patient was delivered.

Not long after that particular event I received a 'please explain' from the DCA saying that the shire clerk out at Jundah had reported the incident of my taking off in such poor conditions, by using just the headlights of a few cars and those of the aeroplane, as being unsafe. So I fronted up and dealt with that. But the irony of it all was that not long after, we were called back to Jundah at ten o'clock one night to evacuate someone who'd suffered a heart attack. So it was obviously dark. When we arrived there we discovered that the patient was the same shire clerk who'd put in the complaint to the DCA. And I can tell you, he was very pleased to see us arrive, and this time there was certainly no complaint about my taking off in the dark, aided by just the headlights of a few cars and those of the aeroplane.

Another memorable night-time event occurred at Nockatunga Station, in the south-western corner of Queensland. We were urgently required to fly out there for an evacuation. Of course, when landing an aeroplane it's standard procedure to land into the wind. To that end, as I always did before I left base,

I checked with Nockatunga as to what the wind direction was and the lady there advised me that the wind was 'an easterly'.

By that stage, people were aware of my requirement of using the lights of three cars in a V shape to assist a night-time landing, so that was organised by the time we got out there. The only trouble was that the lady's understanding of 'an easterly' was that the winds were going to the east and not coming from the east. So an easterly is, in actual fact, a wind that is blowing in from the east. Consequently, on her bad advice I found myself landing downwind and rapidly running out of airstrip. And that really put the wind up the 'light keeper' in the car right at the end of the strip. Because as I was trying to pull up the aeroplane, he came to the rapid conclusion that there was no possible way that I could stop before I hit him, so he bailed out of his vehicle, post haste. Yes, he was out of that car in a flash and he took off.

Anyway, fortunately I was able to pull up without incident. But from then on, whenever I was checking the local conditions I made doubly sure that I phrased my questions in such a way that that type of mistake never occurred again.

But back in the days when cars were used quite extensively to act as runway lights, you really did have some close ones. One of the blokes I really enjoyed flying with was Dr George Ellis. George worked with me in Cairns for a couple of years. And there was one particular night that gave him great cause to worry.

There was a child on Hurricane Station who'd been diagnosed with leukaemia. At that stage the child was able to remain at home, though evacuations were needed from time to time when treatment was required. Anyhow, again it was night, but on this occasion the people helping to light the airstrip proved to be a little too enthusiastic, because as we were coming in to land George exclaimed, 'Gee, Phil, those cars are parked pretty damn close together.'

'Yes,' I replied, trying to gauge if I could land between them without losing our wings.

Then, just as we were about to land, an extremely nervous George asked, 'Do you reckon we'll make it?'

'No,' I said, and we ascended at the rate of knots, weaving our way among the hills, which was a great relief to George.

Now, while I'm on about landing in difficult spots: at one stage in the late-70s, the Cairns *Post* reported how I'd landed my Queen Air aeroplane on a, quote, 'winding mountain road, in the Mount Surprise area'. Well, I'd say to that, 'Don't believe everything you read in the newspapers.'

The true story is as follows: a group of lads were driving over to Karumba, in the lower Gulf area, when they rolled their car about fifteen kilometres out of Mount Surprise. It was quite a bad accident and we were told that the boys may well have spinal injuries. Again, George Ellis was the doctor on call and he advised the locals not to move the lads until we arrived.

Naturally, George wanted me to land as near to the accident scene as possible. I'd done a number of road landings over the years, and just as long as the distance between the trees on either side of a reasonably straight stretch of road was sufficient to land the plane, I could see no problem in achieving that. I'd already been in radio contact with the police from Mount Surprise about all this and requested that they organise for the white road-side posts to be removed for approximately 2000 feet, which they did. Consequently, while it may have looked like a very close thing to those on board the Queen Air aeroplane, including poor George, I landed, again, without incident.

Then after getting help to manually turn the aircraft around we were able to taxi back, closer to the accident site. There the boys were treated by George and the nursing sister, who were then able to use the appropriate shifting techniques to prevent possible further spinal injuries. Once again that evacuation demonstrated the versatility of the Queen Air as being the ideal aircraft for RFDS operations.

Though not all landings went so well. Around 1976, with big rains and flooding across north Queensland, we were called out to Gunnawarra Station, which is south-west of Mount Garnet. Tom Atkinson, the son of the owners, was seriously ill and the doctor decided that even though the weather was terrible, Tom needed to be evacuated to Cairns Base Hospital. When we took off at about midday, this time in a Beechcraft Baron, we could see the Barron River had broken its banks and spread across the Smithfield floodplain.

Following a routine flight we landed on a rather damp Gunnawarra airstrip and were met by Vern Atkinson, Tom's father. Tom was loaded onto the aircraft but, as we taxied for take-off, the nose wheel bogged and, in doing so, the wheel-strut was badly bent. We then radioed the engineers in Cairns who suggested we somehow weld the strut in a fixed down position.

Tom was then off-loaded and we all spent the night at Gunnawarra discussing how we'd make the repairs. Being surrounded by practical blokes—myself included—the following morning we took two pieces of angle-iron out to the plane and, by applying weight on the tail, we lifted the nose wheel off the ground and were able to weld the angle iron to brace the strut. With the job now done, Tom was then reloaded and we made the slow and wet journey back to Cairns, with the landing gear fixed down.

As I half-expected, later in the week the DCA contacted me again. I fully appreciated it was a reportable incident. An investigation was launched with lots of questions being asked. But, in the end, the department decided that, although it was an unusual procedure, under the circumstances they decided not to prosecute. So no further action was taken against me, as pilot in command. And that was another run-in with the DCA.

Another beautiful Atkinson property was the Valley of Lagoons, at the headwaters of the Burdekin River. We conducted regular monthly clinics there so we were well known to the owners. On one occasion we were called there after a mustering accident involving Mark Atkinson, the son of Ivy and Bob, from Glen Eagle. Mark was in a bad way with a broken pelvis and other injuries. This time I was in the King Air and again rain had been falling, which made the airstrip quite a challenge. We landed fine but then, as we taxied, the plane became bogged and we needed to be very practical in solving the problem. So, together with the owner, we used a tractor to tow the aircraft out onto firm land and this second time the take-off went without a hitch. Anyhow, the DCA didn't find out about that one and so there was no further mention of the incident.

Then, no doubt you've heard many stories about having to clear the airstrip of stock such as horses, cattle or sheep, and, of course, there's the ones about kangaroos or emus hopping in front of the aeroplane and being chopped up. But I very much doubt if you've heard of anything like this happening: late one afternoon we took off from the Aboriginal settlement of Kowanyama to go to Pormpuraaw settlement, where we were to run another clinic. Pormpuraaw would only be half an hour's flight from Kowanyama, maybe less. Anyhow, we were up at about 1500 feet, doing the circuit area of Kowanyama, when there came this terrible 'bang!'. Oh, I can tell you, it shook up everyone in the aircraft, me included.

Then, when I looked out the starboard or the right-hand side of the aircraft there, much to my surprise, I saw the backside of an eagle. On further investigation, the rest of his body was embedded in the leading edge of the wing. The poor thing had been happily free-wheeling through a beautiful day, not looking where it was going, and the next thing, 'bang', it'd flown into the wing of the aeroplane, and that's where it stuck. As you might imagine, the wind resistance caused by this body being embedded in the wing disrupted the airflow, which in turn caused the aircraft to veer to the right. There was no hope for the poor bird I'm afraid but, luckily, still being in the circuit area, I decided to land back at Kowanyama, which I did safely and much to the relief of everyone on board. A number of photos were then taken of this magnificent bird, which had a wing-span of over eight feet.

But of course not all the things that happened were caused by external influences. Some disasters happened on board. Such an event I remember only too well. We were called to Killarney Station, in the centre of Cape York, to evacuate a seventeen-year-old who'd broken his ankle while riding a motorbike. It turned out that the lad was the nephew of the owners and was out there holidaying from town. And this young 'townie' had primed himself to the absolute for his 'bush holiday' by giving his image a complete 'manly' overhaul. Oh, this lad was dressed in all his new, and obviously expensive, gear, which were obviously much prized by the lad; you know, the flash RM Williams riding boots, the moleskin trousers, the chequered bush shirt, the lot.

Anyhow, after we arrived the doctor wanted to examine the broken ankle. But because of the swelling they were unable to remove the boot so they had to cut off the expensive RMs. That was the first dent to the lad's new, and expensive, image. Then after his RMs had been cut off, the doctor wanted to get a decent look at the other injuries, so then the precious trousers were cut off. Apart from being in considerable pain the patient was now also severely distressed at realising that this 'manly' image of his was being slowly cut from him and that his 'bush holiday' was coming to a rapid and disastrous end. But more was to follow. Because, amid much screaming, the lad was finally settled onto the stretcher and loaded onto the plane. Then, as we took off for our two-hour flight, the young frightened patient called out, 'I'm gonna shit myself.'

'No, you'll be all right,' replied the extremely patient doctor.

'I won't,' came the loud cry from the lad, as the most shocking smell pervaded the cabin of the aircraft.

'Bush holiday' well and truly over. 'Manly' image completely and utterly destroyed.

Through a Child's Eyes

Now, here's a little ditty for you, and one that's quite cute in its way. It's all to do with how people see things, children in particular. This happened on Killarney Station, which is somewhat north of the Pinnacles, in Queensland, around the Cape York Peninsula region. Now, the people from Killarney Station and the Royal Flying Doctor Service in Queensland had just arranged for the RFDS to begin flying in there on a regular basis to run medical clinics. So, of course, we'd never been to Killarney before. Anyway, we'd arranged that our aircraft was to come in to the station, I think it was at something like ten o'clock in the morning, on such and such a day.

Anyhow, all during the day before we were due to fly out there, and even more so as it got towards nightfall, the family from Killarney were getting pretty excited about our arrival, especially the daughter, who was a young girl of about eleven years of age. So, as the day progressed into night her excitement about the grand occasion built to such an extent that she was almost beside herself. If you could imagine, it was a bit like the grand anticipation of Father Christmas coming the next day. She was forever asking her parents, 'When's the Flying Doctor coming?' and 'How long will it be before the Flying Doctor gets here?'

Now, how they finally got the girl to bed on the night before our arrival, I don't know. And I don't think she even slept a wink. That's how excited she was at the prospect of seeing the Flying Doctor arrive. Then she was up and dressed at about six o'clock the next morning, and wanting to go down to the airstrip.

'Look,' her mother said, 'just leave it a while.'

Anyway, the young girl left it to about eight o'clock, until she could wait no longer, and so then she wandered down to the airstrip by herself, there to stand gazing up into the skies.

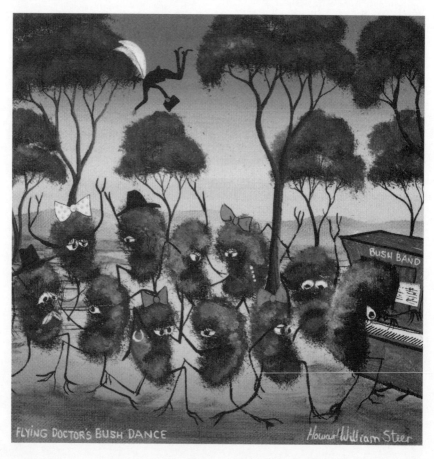

FLYING DOCTOR'S BUSH DANCE   Howard William Steer

At about 9.45 am the mother came down to join her. And the little girl, you know, by this stage she could hardly control herself at the prospect of the Flying Doctor arriving. It was just beyond her.

So the mother and the daughter, there they are, the seconds ticking by and they're looking into the heavens in great anticipation. Then as ten o'clock approached they see this tiny, little speck in the sky and, just at the sight of this speck, this little girl's eyes are becoming the size of saucers. She's just so excited. 'Look, Mummy. Look, Mummy,' she calls, 'it's the Flying Doctor.'

Then as this little speck gradually gets larger and larger and the aeroplane comes more clearly into sight, the little girl's mouth falls open and she looks at her mother in great disgust and disbelief and she grumbles, 'That's not the Flying Doctor, Mummy. It can't be. That's just an ordinary old aeroplane.'

And so, in her childlike imagination, this little girl truly believed that the Flying Doctor was a real doctor, with wings and all, who was going to fly into Killarney Station. And of course Howard William Steer, the great artist of Broken Hill, always paints the Flying Doctor that way: depicting a person, with wings attached, flying through the sky, holding the doctor's bag.

Too Close

I've been with the Flying Doctor Service for nineteen years now and, even still, it's very difficult at times to separate the nurse part of you from the heart and soul person. I guess a good example of that would be when there was a big bus accident out of Coober Pedy, the opal mining place up in the north of South Australia. A group of kids were on a school excursion from Melbourne and about thirty or forty of them were taken to Coober Pedy which, of course, overwhelmed their hospital's resources. Now, I'm not sure just how many injured kids we ended up ferrying out to Adelaide, but we had three aeroplanes working up there. They even flew a plane over from Broken Hill to help out on that one, too. So, it was a big accident.

But in cases like that you always feel for the parents, because no matter how hard you try, sometimes you just can't neglect the mother inside you. And the thing that got to me was that these Melbourne kids were the same age as my own children. And there they were, they'd gone off on a fun school holiday, like most kids do, but, yeah, they ended up in an horrific accident like that. Oh, there were a lot of routine injuries but there were also a few really critically serious ones as well.

So yeah, it took me a long time to come to terms with that. Though, an odd thing happened about that accident because some years later, after we'd moved down to Adelaide, I did an interview for a local newspaper and during that interview they asked me, 'What's been the worst thing you've ever been involved in?' So I mentioned that accident, out at Coober Pedy, and I told them why. Then the night after the newspaper article came out there was a knock on my front door and it was the young lady who owned the house across the road from us.

'Guess what?' she said. 'I was one of the kids who were involved in that bus accident.'

So yeah, that was great, because she told me how some of them had got on and what they were doing, further down the track. So you never know, do you? She was a virtual stranger, just someone you'd say 'hello' to in the street or whatever, and she turned out to be one of the kids we helped that particular night out at Coober Pedy.

But no, to be honest, you don't always survive emotionally intact. Sometimes you're just too close to it all and you get very hurt. Really, one of the reasons I left Port Augusta was that I was starting to pick up people I knew. Some I'd even known when they were babies and I'd seen them grow up, and that was devastating because sometimes they'd suffered indescribable injuries and sometimes they were even killed. So, yes, it became hard, very hard.

Another accident that I found quite emotionally difficult started out when we were on our way up to Mintabie one time. Originally that was for a routine pick-up so we didn't have a doctor with us, because on the more straightforward trips like that you don't need one. So there was just the pilot and myself and we were diverted to Oodnadatta, which is north of Coober Pedy. There'd been a vehicle rollover involving eight people and they were being brought into town by locals, just as we landed. Anyhow, it turned out to be a family that both my husband and I knew very well. Some had even been at school with our children.

But what made it even more difficult was that, other than having to deal with the emotions of knowing these people, basically, to start with there was just myself and two other nurses, plus a man and a woman from Oodnadatta, to attend to these eight people. And a number of them were critically injured and one died before any other help arrived.

Anyhow, we worked on these people for three hours before a retrieval team got in Oodnadatta. The retrieval doctor on that occasion was Fred Gilligan. Fred was lovely. He was just wonderful. As it transpires he went on to be a board member of the RFDS. Yeah, he's just a darling. I fell in love with him that night.

But as you might be able to imagine, with only the three of us there to start with, trying to deal with eight critical patients, stuck out in the bush in a small 'cottage-hospital' well, we were under a huge amount of stress and pressure. We had no x-rays, we had nothing, and we were trying to do the very best we possibly could. So you couldn't really expect us to give the same care as a large city hospital would.

But obviously that's what they expected down in Adelaide. Because after we'd got to the Royal Adelaide Hospital and handed our patients over, I walked outside and discovered that some of the paperwork or something was still in my pocket. Of course, you wouldn't do that these days. But anyway, when I went back to hand it in, one of the Adelaide doctors was going on to Fred Gilligan about the level of care that the patients had received, pre-hospital. And, on top of everything else, what with knowing these people and working under almost impossible conditions, that really hurt, you know. Really hurt.

But Fred stuck up for us. He told them straight out, 'You just have no idea what you're talking about. This was an absolutely horrific accident and those people were working in the most unbelievably difficult conditions.'

So I just thought, Good on you, Fred. I love you. At least you understand what it's like.

Watch What You Say

Just off the bat, I tell you what: you've got to be very, very careful what you say when you're around people who are unconscious, because they can recall things. It's like when someone's in a coma. The best thing to do is to just sit there and chat away to them because quite often, on some subconscious level or other, they can hear you. In cases like that, it's beneficial to the patient. Then, of course, within the Flying Doctor Service there's the other side to it where, particularly if there's been an accident or if there's a fatality where a child is involved, you just don't talk about it anywhere around anyone who's unconscious, especially if it happens to be the parents.

But one, which was a bit of a scream, was when a pilot of ours was doing a retrieval out of Peterborough, in central South Australia. It could've been a road accident, though I'm not sure. But it was out of the old Peterborough airstrip and he was flying the Chieftain and by the time they were ready to take off, he had quite a load. You know, on a trip like that there's not only the retrieval team and the patient but they also carry a lot of extra gear.

Anyhow, the patient was unconscious and because the pilot had so much weight on board, even though he'd done all his calculations, he was still just a little concerned that he didn't have quite enough airstrip to take off. Like, he was sure but not quite one hundred and ten per cent sure, if you catch my meaning. And so as he was starting to roll down the runway, this pilot turned back to the retrieval team and he remarked, pretty much tongue-in-cheek, 'When I yell out, I want you all to take a deep breath so I can get this thing airborne.'

Anyway, later on in hospital, when the patient gained consciousness, some part of him remembered that remark. And when he made enquiries he was told that, yes, in fact the Peterborough airstrip wasn't the most suitable for a retrieval like that and the Flying Doctor Service had mentioned the situation to the authorities, and his particular case was mentioned. Then, after he recovered, he was so grateful to the RFDS that he was the one who instigated the airstrip being moved to a better location and he was also the one responsible for it getting lengthened. I think the old one used to be north-east of Peterborough, out near the meatworks, and the new one's to the south of Peterborough. So that was one of the rare cases where the spoken word around an unconscious patient actually did do some good.

Then I had an incident with a nurse once. It didn't turn out funny, but I thought it was at the moment, though maybe that's just because of my odd sense of 'pilot's' humour. I went to Kadina one time with a nurse. It was in the Chieftain again. So we took off, then, because I couldn't get the green light to come on to give the okay that all was right with the main undercarriage, I decided to return to Adelaide. Really, in a situation like that, in your mind you're fully convinced that it's simply a micro-switch fault. But of course if the worst came to the worst and we did have undercarriage problems, well, it was best to come back to Adelaide and land, because Adelaide Airport has all the fire facilities and the emergency services and so forth.

Anyhow, as we were coming back to Adelaide, coming in to land on runway one and two, from the Gulf, I briefed the nurse on the evacuation of the aircraft. See, as the pilot, it's your job to calm everyone down so they can deal with the emergency. Then, once they're calm, you can go about briefing yourself so that you're also better able to deal with the situation.

But anyway, this nurse kept on asking me question after question and I was getting to the stage where I could hardly think myself. Then as we were coming in on final landing and we were getting in on short-final landing, she said, 'What's the worst that could possibly happen here?'

By this time I was getting a little bit sick of all these queries so I replied in a more-or-less flippant manner, 'Well, the worst thing that could happen is that we crash and burn.'

She just fell into complete silence then and I didn't think any more about it because I was concentrating on the job at hand. So we landed and everything went okay and I taxied back to the hanger and went and spoke to the engineers about the problem. After I'd finished doing that, another pilot came up to me and said, 'What did you do, or say, to the nurse? She's down in the back room in tears.'

And I said, 'Oh God, sorry. I know what it is. I told her that we were going to "crash and burn".'

So I had to go down and console her about it. But, you see, I said it straight off the bat. As a pilot, during your training you're taught to focus in an emergency and delete any of those unnecessary peripheral interferences. So it meant nothing to me, you know, but she asked the question and in the worst case scenario that was the worst thing that could possibly happen—that we would 'crash and burn'. I mean, naturally you don't want that to happen. But, anyway, that's what I said and she took it very seriously.

So you do have to be careful what you say around people, even if they are conscious. And, off the top of my head, that's all I can think of at the moment.

West of the Cooper

There was an old grazier; for the sake of the story we'll call him Arthur. Well, old Arthur lived out west of the Cooper, around the border area of south-western Queensland and north-eastern South Australia. The name of the station just escapes me for the moment so we'll just stick with 'west of the Cooper'.

Now, what you've got to realise here is that a lot of these old fellers who live out in those remote parts of this wide brown land of ours have probably never been out of the bush. So you can imagine that some of them are probably not quite as academically educated as some of us. In fact, some of them can't even read or write. Mind you, that doesn't make them any less of a person. It's just the way it is.

But old Arthur had a cardiac condition and he needed to go and see a specialist, so I gave him a referral to go and see a specialist in Brisbane. Brisbane was the town of his choice. It wasn't an emergency or anything, it was just routine, so he got on a commercial flight from Windorah and headed off to Brisbane. It was all a new experience for him because, firstly, I don't think he'd ever been on a commercial aeroplane before and, secondly, to my recollection, he'd never been to Brisbane.

When the specialist saw old Arthur, he reckoned that there wasn't much more to be done other than what I'd already recommended he do. That was reassuring to me. But a few weeks later the specialist sent Arthur an account and on the account you've got the Medicare item number which was, we'll say for argument's sake, 'Item No. 76'.

Anyway, when old Arthur looked at this account, he couldn't make head nor tail of it. But he did see this No. 76. And you know how all the drugs in the RFDS medical chest are labelled by numbers, well, when old Arthur saw this No. 76 he thought, 'Well, that specialist feller must want me to take No. 76 out of the RFDS medical kit.'

Then when I was out there, the next month, I saw old Arthur and he said to me, 'Gees,' doctor,' he said, 'that number seventy-six didn't do me a scrap of good.'

'What do you mean?' I said.

'Well,' he said, 'look here; on my account it's got number seventy-six.'

And that's when I discovered that old Arthur had, in actual fact, mixed up the Medicare number with the item number in the RFDS medical kit and had been taking some sort of anti-fungal medication.

The next story also comes from out west of the Cooper.

I got a call one evening—it was after last light—to go out to South Galway Station. One of the ringers there was in some sort of strife. So, you know, we asked them to put out their flares and one thing and another and I told them that we'd be in touch with an ETA as soon as we got in the air. There was the pilot, a nurse and myself.

Then, when we called through to South Galway Station with the ETA, they told us that there were severe thunderstorms in the area. Now, thunderstorms are a real hazard to flying. First, they can create incredible turbulence. Second, with these being dirt airstrips, they can turn to mud in an instant.

Anyway, the pilot said, 'Oh well, we'll just continue on and see what happens.'

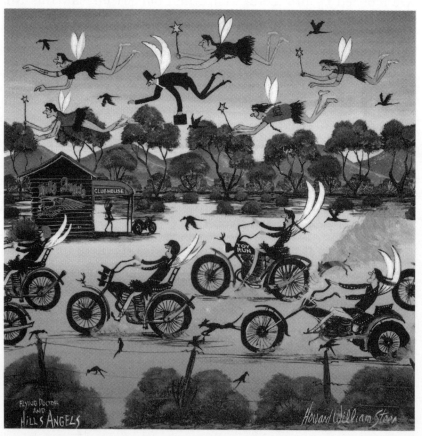

So we continued on. But then just as we arrived over South Galway Station so did the thunderstorm. Oh, it was blowing a beauty and it was raining like crazy. This, in turn, caused most of the flares, which they'd lit for us along the runway, to be either blown out or doused in the rain—one or the other. But fortunately the pilot knew the strip quite well and he reckoned that by using the flashes of lightning as a guide, he could see just enough of the airstrip to land the aeroplane. And that's what he did: he put the plane down on the strip by using the flashes of lightning, along with the few flairs that still remained alight. Some of these pilots do amazing things, and that was just one of them.

Anyhow, luckily for us they'd already brought the injured ringer out to the strip, which saved precious time. But even still, with it now raining cats and dogs and the dirt strip rapidly turning greasy, I quickly assessed the situation and decided that if I didn't open the door, put the injured ringer on board, quickly tie him down, shut the door again and get out of there, we'd end up being stuck on the strip—bogged. All patients in stretchers have to be tied down. It's procedure.

So we did that. We loaded this ringer as quickly as we could. Then we tied him down in the stretcher, shut the door, and I told the pilot to get going, which he did, and we took off safely.

But, of course, with this thunderstorm going on all around us, the turbulence was something incredible. As I assessed the patient, we were being tossed around like anything. So

I thought, Well, the first thing I need to get into him is an intravenous cannula and a drip.

So I put a tourniquet on him and I literally threw the cannula into his arm like a dart, sort of thing, and it happened to hit a vein. Then I looked over at my nurse, fully expecting her to pass me the drip set, only to find that she had her head stuck in a sick bag. Well, it was all too much for me and I then also had to grab a bag. So there I was, being tossed around in the turbulence, while trying to keep a bag over my face, with one hand holding the drip into the ringer's arm and the other hand trying to put the giving-set into the drip.

And that's when the ringer looked up at us and he said, 'I think I'm probably the best of all of yer.'

What If

We used the Flying Doctor Service in 1980 when my daughter, Megan, got bitten by a redback spider. At the time we were caretaking out at Mt Barnett Station, in the Kimberley area of Western Australia, while the owners went away for holidays over the wet season. Megan was about six years old, in Year 1. Her dad, Colin, was playing guitar and she was sitting on a cyclone bed. You know those old cyclone beds, the pipe ones with the hollow legs with the wire mesh on top. Well, Megan was sitting on one of those and she said, 'Daddy, something just bit me.'

Then, when Colin looked down the hollow pipe, he saw a redback spider sitting in there. So we called the Flying Doctor. That was at about one o'clock and they said they'd attempt to get there by three o'clock. In the meantime, of course, we had to try and keep Megan calm and also try and keep ourselves calm.

Anyhow, with it being the wet season, the river was in full flood and the airstrip was on the other side of the river from where the homestead was. So then Colin and I, we had to row Megan across the flooded river in a little dinghy. The distance was probably, oh, a couple of hundred yards or so; you know, from about here, where I'm sitting, right over there to the corner of the road. Yes, that'd make it about two hundred yards or so, and when we finally got to the airstrip there was a new doctor on the plane. The funny part about that was—and, mind you, it wasn't too funny at the time—when we got on the plane, there he was, this doctor, busily looking up some book or other trying to find out what you're supposed to do with someone who'd been bitten by a redback spider.

And I thought, Oh, this looks real good, this does.

But that was the thing in those days with the RFDS because back in 1980 they didn't have their own doctors. Back then, the Flying Doctor Service was using the local hospital doctors. And you get a lot of turnover up in the Kimberley and the frustration with that was that, when a new doctor arrived, quite often they wouldn't be familiar with RFDS procedure and, for that matter, a lot of them weren't even familiar with the contents of the RFDS medical chest. You know, what number equates to what medicine you're supposed to take for whatever the ailment or problem you have. Worse still, if these doctors had just graduated from Perth or wherever they probably didn't even know that the RFDS medical chest existed, if you know what I mean.

Anyhow, I must say that it was a great relief to have the plane arrive and take us back to Derby. But Megan wasn't given anything until we got into hospital. Even then she had to wait because it wasn't until six o'clock that another doctor came in and said, 'Has she been given the anti-venom yet?'

'What're you talking about?' I asked.

'Oh,' he said, 'if it was my kid, she'd be given the anti-venom straight away.'

Okay then, I thought, if it's a doctor saying that, surely they'll do it soon.

But still nothing, and Megan was just left to lie there in the hospital bed. And though she wasn't all that sick, you could see the bite mark and her leg had become quite swollen. But I didn't know anything about spider bites. I didn't know how sick she was supposed to be.

Anyway, this all happened just before the people we were caretaking for at Mt Barnett Station—John and Bronwyn Tiddy—were going to go back out there. So they were in Derby and John Tiddy came into the hospital and I remember the nurse suddenly appearing with the first injection. And Megan, all her life she just hated injections. Oh, she just hated injections.

Then the nurse held up the needle and said, as easy going as anything, 'We're just going to give you this for pain.'

And John Tiddy knew all about Megan's hatred of needles and you could see that he was just about to have a go at the nurse, because, you know, Megan hadn't been given any warnings that she was even going to have a needle. Anyhow, the nurse went ahead and gave Megan the needle for the pain. Then, just when Megan was starting to get over the trauma of that, they came back in and said they had to give her a few more test shots for the anti-venom. In the end, I think they gave her three needles all up. And each time the nurse came back brandishing a needle, Megan was getting more and more upset and John Tiddy's getting madder and madder.

And, well, the reason why John was the only male there with me was because Colin was still out at Mt Barnett. They couldn't take Colin on the plane because they didn't have enough room for him. They only took me and Megan. And that was quite funny too, actually, because I found out later that after we'd flown out, when Colin had started rowing back to the homestead the dinghy got caught in a whirlpool or something and he ended up being taken a fair way down the river before he could get himself onto land again. And when he finally managed to do that, he had to walk all the way back to the homestead. So there was another drama going on.

Anyway, they gave Megan the anti-venom and everything and then of course from that day on she had to wear a Medic-Alert bracelet. See, back in those days the anti-venom was given in a horse serum base and she had to wear the bracelet to alert everyone that if she was bitten again and had to have a second dose of the anti-venom, they had to watch her very carefully because the second dose could well bring on an anaphylactic reaction. An anaphylactic reaction is a full-on, life-threatening allergic reaction where, you know, you start swelling up and you can't breathe and all that sort of stuff. It's like having a heart attack. Of course, these days all the anti-venom's given in synthetic bases so Megan doesn't have to worry about that any more.

So, you know, for all the fuss and worry that it caused later, I really think that Megan would have probably been better off not having the anti-venom. We discovered afterwards that she was most probably bitten by the less venomous male redback because she didn't end up getting the full-blown symptoms of a spider bite, you know, with the vomiting and the heavy sweating and all that sort of stuff. Megan only had a swollen leg and a tiny red area around the bite. So in fact she didn't really need the injections or the anti-venom or anything like that.

Then, of course, after she was injected with the anti-venom in a horse serum base it caused us a lot of anxiety because we were always worried about what would happen if she got bitten by something again and she had to have another anti-venom injection. You know, whether she'd have an anaphylactic reaction and all that. So it was all very scary because living in that country you always think, God, what if she's bitten by an extremely venomous snake like a King Brown and she has to go through it all again? So that's the end of that story.

Glory, Glory—The Flying Doctor Song

Verse 1

A ringer lay dying out in a stock camp

Thrown from his horse and trampled about

In a feverish haze and in sickening pain

He raises his head and then he says

Chorus

Glory, Glory what can it be

There's a sound up on high that only angels can see

Glory, Glory what can it be

The Flying Doctor is coming for me

Verse 2

A child is lost a long way from home

Out in the distance water forms

So she walks and she walks till she stumbles and falls

Then she raises her head ... and she calls

Chorus

Glory, Glory what can it be

There's a sound up on high that only angels can see

Glory, Glory what can it be

The Flying Doctor is coming for me

Bridge

In the footsteps of Flynn these women and men
Give of themselves our faith in their hands
Come every day they're working to spread
A mantle of safety across this wide land

Chorus

Glory, Glory what can it be
There's a sound up on high that only angels can see
Glory, Glory what can it be
The Flying Doctor is coming for me

Verse 3

Out from the Alice a lady moans
Heavy with child and on her own
No chance could there be that the baby be saved
So she raises her head and she prays

Chorus

Glory, Glory what can it be
There's a sound up on high that only angels can see
Glory, Glory what can it be
The Flying Doctor is coming for me

The RFDS Today

The Royal Flying Doctor Service of Australia (RFDS) is a not-for-profit charitable organisation that provides free aero-medical emergency and comprehensive healthcare services to people who live, work and travel in regional and remote Australia.

RFDS Statistics for the year ended 30th June 2009:

- Service area—7,150,000 km².
- Patients attended—274,237 (daily average—751). That figure includes patients at clinics, patients transported, immunisations and telehealth.
- Aero-medical evacuations—36,832 (daily average 101). That figure includes interhospital transfers.
- Healthcare Clinics—14,004 (daily average 38).
- Distance flown—23,923,440 kilometres (daily average 65,544 km).
- Number of landings—71,770 (daily average 197)
- Telehealth—85,290 (daily average 234)
- Number of aircraft—53.
- RFDS Bases—21. A RFDS Base is a health facility that houses an aircraft and provides health services.

- RFDS Health Facilities—5. A RFDS Health Facility is a health facility that does not have an aircraft but provides health services.
- Other facilities—10.* Other facilities include marketing, fundraising and public relations as well as the National Office.
- Staff—964. That figure includes 297 part-time and casual staff.

*Source—Royal Flying Doctor Service website.

How You Can Help

The RFDS relies on generous contributions from individuals, community groups, business and the corporate sector as well as funding provided by the Commonwealth, state and territory governments to help meet the costs associated with running a 24-hour emergency and comprehensive healthcare service.

The RFDS relies on your help to:
- Buy vital medical equipment
- Purchase and outfit aircraft (at a cost of more than $8 million each)
- Develop a range of outback and rural health initiatives.

There are many ways in which you, your workplace, community group or school can help the Flying Doctor. By raising money and awareness about the work of the RFDS, you are helping to save lives.

To help our service and save lives in the outback you can:
- Donate online at www.flyingdoctor.net
- Become an RFDS supporter
- Leave a bequest
- Fundraise for the RFDS
- Join an RFDS Workplace Giving initiative

- Volunteer your time or expertise
- Organise an RFDS speaker
- Offer corporate support
- Make a purchase through our online shop
- Send a cheque (made payable to the Royal Flying Doctor Service of Australia) to:

  Australian Council of the RFDS

  Level 8, 15–17 Young Street

  Sydney NSW 2000

  Phone the RFDS on 02-8259 8100 or 1800 467 435

  All donations of $2 and above are tax deductible.

Future Projects

Great Australian Outback School Days Stories

If you have a story or two to tell about your outback school days, please contact me—**before June 2012**—via my email address of bill@billswampymarsh.com or ring (08) 8132 0215 to organise a time for an interview.

Please note that we **<u>do not</u>** accept written submissions.

All stories are written from interviews that have been recorded with the contributors.

All stories are shown to the contributors for their checking and okay before being submitted for the possible inclusion in the book.